CURATIVE EURYTHMY

First English Edition, Rudolf Steiner Press, London 1983

Translated from shorthand reports unrevised by the lecturer.
The original German text is published in the Complete Edition
of the works of Rudolf Steiner entitled, *Heileurythmie*
(No. 315 in the Bibliographical Survey 1961).

This English edition is published in agreement with the
Rudolf Steiner Nachlassverwaltung, Dornach, Switzerland.
This translation by Kristina Krohn in collaboration with
Dr. Anthony Degenaar has been made from the German
Fourth Edition, 1981.

British Library Cataloguing in Publication Data

Steiner, Rudolf
   Curative eurythmy
   1. Dance therapy
   2. Movement therapy
   I. Title   II. Heileurythmie. *English*
   615.8'2   RC489.D3

   ISBN 0-85440-398-1

Printed and bound in Great Britain at
The Camelot Press Ltd, Southampton

CURATIVE EURYTHMY

RUDOLF STEINER

Eight Lectures
given in Dornach, Switzerland
between 12th and 18th of April, 1921,
and in Stuttgart, Germany
on October 28th, 1922.

Rudolf Steiner Press
London

THE PUBLICATION OF RUDOLF STEINER'S LECTURES

The foundation of anthroposophically orientated Spiritual Science is laid in the works which were written and published by Rudolf Steiner (1861-1925). At the same time Dr.Steiner held numerous lectures and courses both for the general public and for members of the Theosophical (later Anthroposophical) Society in the years between 1900 and 1924. It was not his original wish to have these lectures published which were without exception of a spontaneous nature and conceived as "oral communications not intended for print". However, after an increasing number of incomplete and erroneous listeners' transcripts had been printed and circulated, he found it necessary to have the notes regulated. He entrusted this task to Marie von Sivers. She was made responsible for the choice of stenographers, the supervision of their transcripts and the necessary revision of texts before publication. As Rudolf Steiner was only in a very few instances able to correct the notes himself his reservation in respect to all publications of his lectures must be taken into account: "Errors occurring in transcripts which I myself have been unable to revise will just have to be tolerated."

In Chapter 35 of his autobiography, Rudolf Steiner expounds on the relationship between his lectures for members which were initially only circulated internally and his public writings. The relevant text is printed at the end of this volume. What is expressed there also applies to the lecture courses directed towards a restricted audience already familiar with the principles of Spiritual Science.

After Marie Steiner's death (1867-1948) the editing of a "Complete Works of Rudolf Steiner" was commenced according to her directions. The volume at hand constitutes a part of this complete edition.

iv

CONTENTS

FOREWORD TO THE ENGLISH EDITION

There are many difficulties involved in translating the curative eurythmy course. In order to remain as close to Rudolf Steiner's meaning as possible, it was agreed to make as literal a translation as was necessary. It was therefore clear from the beginning that the text could not read like an English composition. In the German, one has of course to do with the spoken word, which is less clearly formulated than a written text. Furthermore, in this course Steiner develops concepts which are being formulated for the first time. His difficulty in finding the means to convey these ideas adequately is evident to begin with in the analogies he brings, which are in themselves complicated, and, what is here more important, in the way he bends and reshapes the German language to follow the contours of the thoughts. His intent is often more evident in the sound of the words and their sequence rather than in their meaning, as was justified in speaking to eurythmists. No attempt has been made to spare the English reader the work of following Steiner by translating intellectually what we understand his meaning to be. Sentences which are difficult to understand will on comparison generally be found to be equally difficult in German. Where an uncertainty arose in the German text it has been left as such in the English.

It is important to attempt to follow the invisible being of this course which is expressed only in its barest substance by the text. Repeated readings of the lectures will reveal an inner plan which is not at first apparent. The course outlines the inner structure of curative eurythmy and thus in its own way that of the human being.

The German pronunciation of the alphabet has been retained throughout as it is assumed that all practitioners of curative eurythmy will already be familiar with this usage.

Dortmund, West Germany
December 1982

Kristina Krohn

SYNOPSIS OF LECTURES

work in the consonant and their effect. The speech-physiological processes that accompany the speaking of vowels and their use in curative eurythmy. The inner connection between the formative tendencies in speaking and eurythmic movements carried out for curative purposes. Movement in the will and movement in the intellect. The losing of the formative quality of language by the intellect as being the inner cause of illness. Eurythmy brings the formative quality and the will element back into language.

spiritually-orientated physiological element. Example of a recitation of Goethe's poem "Über allen Gipfeln ist Ruh...", performed in eurythmy first with the vowels and then with the consonants. The essence of listening. Listening is a condition similar to sleep, a gentle imagining. The ether movements of the person who is asleep or who is listening are made visible by the physical body in eurythmy. Doing vowels and consonants alternately in eurythmy stimulates the forces of growth.

curative eurythmy the curative process arises through intensive co-operation between doctor and curative eurythmist. A thorough diagnosis is a prerequisite of curative eurythmy. The effect of speech and curative eurythmy on the organism (examples of exercises). Human organs should be observed in their polarity: centrifugal and centripetal dynamics. Sensitivity and an artistic disposition are essential for being active as a curative eurythmist. Curative eurythmy must be backed up by actual therapy. Curative eurythmy is more important than massage because it has an effect on all the members of man's being. Gym and curative eurythmy. Experience in curative eurythmy gained through practice. Not to be used in the case of fractures or carcinomas. A warning against dilettantism. Soul-spiritual element added to existing physiology and anatomy. Shallow criticism must not be tolerated. Opponents and misunderstandings.

LECTURE 1

Dornach, April 12, 1921

In these afternoon hours I wish to present the first seeds of a curative eurythmy. Today we will have a sort of introduction, and what we gain from it we will develop into definite forms in the days following. First of all I want to draw attention to some basic matters. What has been practised up until now is eurythmy as art; and as such it should be concomitantly accepted as the eurythmy pedagogically and didactically suited for children, since what has been developed until now as eurythmy is in every way drawn out of the formation of the healthy human being. We will see that certain points of contact appear, by means of which it will be possible to distil a hygienic-therapeutic discipline from the eurythmic, and how certain artistic forms transform themselves in one direction or another to become what can be called a sort of curative eurythmy.

It will, of course, be essential to emphasize that artistic eurythmy — which is in essence the expression of that element inherent in the formation and in the tendencies to movement of the human body — is that which must be adjudged correct for the development of the human organism as soul, spirit and body, even as it is appropriate for visual presentation. However, one can also work towards a curative eurythmy which will be of extensive use in the treatment of various chronic and acute conditions, but which will prove to be especially important and to the point in those cases specifically where we attempt to treat impending sicknesses and tendencies to sickness, prophylactically through eurythmy. Here is the point at which the didactic-pedagogical element in eurythmy flows gradually over into the hygienic-therapeutic.

However, for those who wish to practise artistic eurythmy, I want to specifically emphasize that they will have to forget in the most thorough fashion what they have acquired in these hours when they do artistic eurythmy. Then precisely in this area one must maintain a strict separation between those goals which one pursues in hygiene and therapeutics and that artistic quality which one must strive to attain in eurythmy. And anyone who persists in mixing the two will first of all ruin his artistic ability in eurythmy and secondly find himself unable to achieve anything of importance in respect to its hygienic-therapeutic element. Apart from this it will be necessary to acquire certain physiological knowledge — which will transform itself into a sort of feeling for the processes forming the human organism — in order to apply the hygienic-therapeutic side of eurythmy practically, as we will see in the following lectures.

Now, having given this preface, I would like to speak more specifically about what may be considered the basis for human eurythmy itself since it appears to me to be pertinent to the goals we wish to attain. If one wishes to understand what eurythmy in its most varied aspects is, one must first of all gain a certain understanding of the human larynx. We will come to know the other vocal organs of man precisely through the course of our exercises relating to it. But the first thing which we must obtain will be a certain knowledge of the human larynx and its importance for the human organization in general. There is much too strong a tendency to regard each human organ as a thing unto itself. That isn't the case, however. That is not how a human organ is. Every human organ is a member of the organization as a whole and, at the same time, a metamorphic variation of certain other organs. Basically, every self-contained human organ is a metamorphosis of other self-contained human organs. Nevertheless, the case is that certain human organs and groups of organs prove to carry this metamorphic character more exactly within them, more precisely, I would like to say, and others less precisely.

An example of an organ where one can penetrate through that one organ into the essence of the human organism solely through a properly understood metamorphosis is the larynx. Recall from your anatomical and physiological knowledge how peculiarly the human larynx is formed.

What I wish to convey can be grasped only through Goetheanistic contemplation of the human larynx. However, if you will make the effort to attain to this Goetheanistic contemplation of the organs involved to which we will now direct our attention, you will see that it is possible. If you take the larynx first of all as an upwards directed extension of the windpipe, you will discover when you study its forms that it may be characterized as a reversed, a from front-to-back reversed piece of the human organism; from another place, another piece of the human organization turned around. Picture to yourself the back of the human head, including the auricular parts, and think of what you are picturing to yourself as the back of the human head, including the auricular parts — insofar as these are localized in this part of man — excluding the frontal lobe* for the moment, and extending downwards so that it becomes the human ribcage with its vertebrae, including the beginnings of the ribs which have the much softer breast bone to the front that falls away altogether lower down. Picture to yourself, then, this less clearly defined — system of organs that I have presented to you: the posterior part of the head including the auditory parts, broadening out into the ribcage below.

And now think of this part somewhat transformed; imagine the diameter of the ribs greatly reduced. Imagine that which is very wide in the ribs, in the ribcage, here transformed into a pipe, the bony material being replaced by cartilage. That part which I isolated as the head, imagine that to be filled out in such a way that the less well filled out parts of the head, were poured out, and then that what is now filled in with thicker tissue were left out; think of that which in the

* Vorderhirn; literally, the frontal lobe of the brain.

3

head is actually filled with a liquid-solid mass replaced. When you imagine this transformation of these parts of the human organism, then you have the metamorphosis of the larynx: the posterior head with the attached ribcage, reversed. The upwards extension into the larynx is truly a sort of posterior head, transformed. It is actually so: the etheric formative forces of the larynx bring about an inversion when we compare them with the formative forces of the aforementioned part of the posterior head with the attached ribcage. Considering the matter etherically, we carry in our breast, in the larynx, a second man, in a manner of speaking, who is, to be certain, in a way rudimentary, but who is in his dispositions, in his beginnings nevertheless at a certain stage of development.

If that which I have just described to you were to be turned around again to its former position so as to appear as the posterior head, then it would, in accordance with the formative forces, of necessity add on those parts of the brain lying further forwards. The tendency to build something similar on is also present in the larynx. The larynx has for this reason the thyroid gland in its neighborhood. What appears in more recent physiology as the peculiar conditions of the thyroid can be understood metamorphically, if you can see a sort of decadent frontal lobe in the thyroid which to a certain extent performs functions taken over from the frontal lobe in the speaking man. The thyroid must co-operate with the frontal lobe. If the thyroid is in any way diseased, you can easily imagine what sort of conditions arise; simply because he has the thyroid, man is organized to use it as an additional organ of thought related more to his breast being.

That which I have designated as etheric formative forces which are at work to bring this second man, who takes up an appositive position in us, into being: — these etheric formative forces are in fact very differentiated. When we breathe and this breathing expresses itself in speaking or singing, when this modified breathing (for from a certain point of view one must call it that) lives as speech or song, then that whole system of organs in man, which I have already indicated as the posterior head continuing down into the breast, is in such inner movement, that this movement experiences its reflexes in the organization of the larynx. So we must picture to ourselves that this whole system — that together with the ear is nothing other than a larynx, only metamorphosed — there is a frontal lobe — calls forth certain effects which are reflected. Thus our larynx performs backwards, in eurythmy, in the form of forces, what we think, feel and so on. This eurythmy really goes on within us. Our larynx eurythmizes; and we have then the assignment to turn around again that which arises sensibly-supersensibly through the reflex-reaction of the larynx, and to make it visible, so that our arms bring to expression that which has already been relayed forth and back again. Thus we have to do here with something which is taken directly from the human organism.

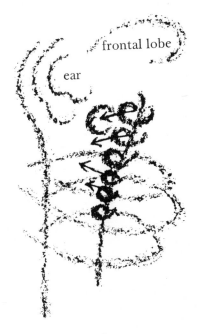

One must make it clear to oneself that we are drawing attention to that organ which like an additional head with a downward extension has been set into the rhythmic system. Our ordinary head, the more or less thoughtful head, has the peculiarity of quieting down what pulses up rhythmically into it through the arachnoidal cavity, which is an extension of the respiratory system. It is by means of the transformation of the movement from below in the rhythmic system into quiet; and by virtue of the fact that a state of balance is reached and stasis is developed out of elements in movement, reciprocally conditioning each other in motion, that thinking is conditioned: through statics arising in the head out of the dynamics.

The reverse is also true: what we develop in the quiet, in the stasis of the head, influences the dynamic of the rhythmic man, to begin with in a retardative manner. The fact is that an unnatural exertion of the soul-spiritual in connection with the head tends to slow down the circulation. A further consequence is that chaotic or sloppy thinking transforms the rhythmic into the arhythmic, changes the natural rhythm which should play in the human rhythmic system into arhythm, even into an antirhythm when it comes to full expression. And if one wishes to understand man, one must observe the connection between the circulatory and respiratory system, and careless, chaotic thought, as well as logical thought. Logical thinking as such carries within it the tendency to slow down the rhythm. Logical thought has the peculiarity of falling out of rhythm. Therefore, the soul-life that wishes to fall into rhythm will try to supercede logic and attempt to frame sentences and verses that follow not syntax, but rhythm in their course. By striving to return to rhythm in poetry, by resisting the enemy of poetry, that is prose (with the exception of rhythmical prose, of course), one tries to become more human. I am not claiming that through logic one's development will tend more towards the animalic; when you wish, you can always imagine that one evolves towards the angelic. But when one strives to turn back from the logical towards the human, one must try to bring into the succession of the syllables and their movement, into the movement of the sounds and into the sentence structure, not that which is demanded by the syntax, but that which the rhythm requires. We must pay heed to the rhythmic man when we want to return to the realm of poetry; we should listen to the head-man when we wish to enter into prose.

This will serve as an indication of the connection which in fact exists between that manifest part of man which I have described and that part which, as a metamorphosis of it, is somewhat concealed. He is there within us, however, this eurythmist who performs as the etheric body of the larynx a distinct eurythmy intimately connected with the normal development of our respiratory system, with our whole circulatory system and, naturally, through the intermediary of the circulatory system even with the metabolic system, as you can surmise from all that I have presented to you.

Now all possible sorts of occasions arise for this very complicated arrangement, this dove-tailing of a forwards- and a backwards-orientated system, to become disjointed. It would be accurate to say that they are properly articulated in only very few people of today's culture. It will be necessary to develop a certain ability to observe this since when the head system, for example, has been so dealt with in childhood that the transgression against the rhythmic system is too great everything possible can develop in later years simply through an irregularity in what I have described. This is precisely because in the case of the human organism, as in an avalanche, small provocations may build up to great effects.

In observing children from this aspect one will find that it is extremely significant to what degree their unconscious living in rhythm predominates in their soul-life over the quieting element of the head organization; for example if this is the case, if the rhythmic system predominates, one must ask oneself if something should not be introduced into

7

the education of the child. If in time the condition appears to be habitual, then something must be done. When, as a result of the anomaly to which I have drawn attention, the child becomes increasingly excited, ever more and more fluttery and one can do nothing with him, one must attempt to bring an iambic element into his whole organization. This can be done by having the child move in such a manner that, in full consciousness — and for that he must have your guidance — he moves first the left arm and the left hand forwards, thereafter the right arm, so that this becomes the more conscious. The child must be aware: that is the first and was the first. Throughout the entire exercise the consciousness must prevail: that was the first and remains the first; it began with the left. One can reinforce the whole affair by having the child walk, stepping out with the left leg and bringing the right leg up to it, so that the leg and foot exercise is added to the hand and arm exercise, but only as a reinforcement, however. The arm exercise is really the essential. If one has the child practise in this iambic manner, as one may call it, one will see that the exercises will calm the fluttery child, the excited child and so on provided they are continued over a sufficiently long period of time.

Out of your knowledge of eurythmy you could describe it thus:* You have the child make half an "A" with the left arm and then complete this half "A" to a whole "A" with the right arm, and so on, so that the child remains in motion and the "A" does not come into being all at once, but as the result of successive movements.

If on the other hand one has a child who is phlegmatic, who doesn't want to take things in — our Waldorf teachers

* The sounds are given throughout the English text as they are written in German: German "a", "ah" as in English "father"; German "e", "a" as in English "say"; German "i", "ee" as in English "feet"; German "ei", "i" as in English "light"; German "au", "ow" as in English "how"; German "eu", "oi" as in English "joy".

know these children well, they can at times bring one to mild despair; they actually hear nothing of what one says to them, everything passes them by — in this case one would do well to treat this child trochaically, that is to say, in just the opposite manner. Naturally one cannot begin with everything all at once; this is an element which has yet to be brought into Waldorf education. One forms the "A" so that the child knows: first the right arm, then the left arm, right arm, left arm and then further that first the right leg is placed in front and the left leg brought up to it; thus one has the arm movements forming the "A" (one after the other) reinforced by the leg and foot movement. One must pay particular attention that these things are done in such a way that they live in the child's consciousness; so that the child is really aware: on one occasion the left arm was the first, on the other the right arm was the first.

You will find that these things present difficulties for an inner understanding if someone is in every way a physiologist in the modern sense and believes that man's whole soul-life is mediated through the nervous system, that is, if you do not know that feeling is mediated by the rhythmic system and the will by the metabolic system, and that only thought formation is mediated by the nervous system. If you do not know these things you will have great difficulty in grasping the significance of what happens in any part of the body, both in respect to the soul-spiritual part and the bodily part of man's being.

The person who has developed an ability to observe knows that when a person has clumsy hand and finger movements and so on, he will exhibit a particular manner of thinking as well which one can compare with what happens in the fingers. It is really extremely interesting to study the connection between the manner in which a person controls the mechanics of the arm and the finger-physiognomy with the way in which he thinks. Then the soul-spiritual qualities which a person portrays proceed from the whole human being, not solely from the brain and nervous tissue. One must learn to understand that one thinks not only with the brain but also with the little finger and the big toe. There is a certain significance in achieving lightness — particularly in the limbs — as this will bring lightness into the soul-life as well. These ideas will only become applicable — as we shall see in the following lectures — when one has the possibility of providing a truly complete school hygiene to accompany the other instruction. It can happen, for example, that a child has the peculiarity of being unable to comprehend geometric figures. He cannot understand a geometric figure by looking at it. However difficult it may be you will do this child a great service when you have him take a small pencil between the big toe and the next toe, hold it and write really proper letters. That is something which carries a certain significance and which points in a fully justified manner to an inter-relationship in man.

Especially in the case of children, one may notice that the three members of the human organization do not snap properly into one another. A really large part of the anomalies of life are due to this improper articulation. To begin with, the children have headaches and at the same time one notices that the digestion is disturbed and so on. The most varied conditions may appear. We will give further indications in this regard in conjunction with other exercises which will be shown in the next days. However, when one is confronted with a situation such as I have described one can achieve a great deal with the child or children through having them do the following exercise: a eurythmic I — as you already know — a eurythmic A and a eurythmic O; but so that the children make the "I" with the whole upper body. For our physician friends I want to emphasize particularly, that what is essential in eurythmy, and that through which one achieves what is essential in artistic eurythmy as well, is not the mere form of the limb in position seen from without, but that which comes into being when the stretching or the bending

10

within the positioned limb is felt. What is felt in the limb is what is important. Assume that you make an "I" with both arms; this "I" will not appear as it should when seen from without if you observe only its line, its content as a form. You must feel concurrently and you can tell by looking at the person — that he feels the stretching power in the I as he does it. Similarly when a person makes an "E", for example, the important thing is not that he does this (crosses the arms), but that he feels: here one limb comes to rest on the other. In this feeling of one limb on the other lies the "E" in reality. And that which one sees in the expression for this sensing of one limb through the other. Then what you do here is no different from what you do when you look. You are continually carrying out an "E" by crossing the axis of the right eye with the axis of the left in order to find a point and so arrive at a crossed line. That is actually "the primeval E". What has been demonstrated here is basically an imitation of it; however, everything in man is a metamorphosis, and this is a perfectly justifiable imitation, as in speaking "E" the larynx carries out exactly the same form to the rear in the etheric.

When you practise this exercise with a child it is necessary that the "I" be done with the upper body, that is to say, the child stretches out his upper body. He feels the whole body stretched. He makes the "A" with his legs and the "O" by moving his arms so. Have the child do the following as quickly as possible in sequence: stretch the upper body vertically, separate the legs, and make the "O" movement with the arms; release and repeat, release and repeat and so on. One can practise such a thing with the children in chorus, of course. However, in principle such exercises should not be practised with the children as a class. Artistic eurythmy and the eurythmy for pedagogic and didactic reasons should be done by a class as a whole, for here children of the same age belong together. In order to make the transition from the usual class eurythmy to these matters related to hygienic-

11

therapeutic eurythmy, one must take those children out of various classes who, due to the peculiarities which I have described — the disharmony of the three members of the human organism — have need of such an exercise, in order to practise with them. One can take them out of the most varied classes and then practise this exercise with those particularly suited for it. That really must be done if one truly wishes to pursue hygienic eurythmy, therapeutic eurythmy, in the school. Thus we are already on the path which as we follow it further will lead us to study certain movements that are actually only metamorphoses of the usual eurythmic movements and to trace their effect on the human organization. The fact is that we have organs in our interior and these organs have certain forms. These forms may be subject to anomalies. The form of each organ stands in a certain relationship to a possible form of movement of the outer man. Therefore the following may be said. Let us assume that some organ, let us say the gall, has the tendency to deformation, a tendency to assume an abnormal form. A form of movement exists which will counteract this tendency. And such is the case with every organ.

It is in this direction that we intend to develop what will follow. What I have given today was meant as an introduction to guide you to the path leading into this subject.

LECTURE 2

Dornach, April 13, 1921

Today I intend to discuss matters related to the vowel element in eurythmy. We need only to recall — as it is known to us through spiritual science — that vowels express more that which lives inwardly in man as feelings, emotions and so on. Consonants describe more that which is outwardly objective. When we remain within the realm of speech, these two statements are valid: vowels, more expression, revelation of the inwardness of feeling; we reveal ourselves to an extent in the vowel, that is to say, we reveal what we feel towards an object. Through the movements which the tongue, the lips and the palate perform, the consonants conform themselves more plastically to the outward forms of objects — as they are spiritually experienced, naturally — and attempt to reconstruct them. And so basically all consonants are more reproductions of the outward form-nature of things. However, one can actually only speak of vowels and consonants in this manner when one has an earlier stage of human evolution in mind in which in fact the evolution of speech was given and in which — since the individual sounds were always to a degree connected with movements of the body — the movement of the whole body and of the limbs as well was self-evident. This connection has been loosened, however, in the course of man's development. Speech was removed more to the interior and the possibilities of movement, of expression through movement, ceased. Today in normal life we speak largely without accompanying our speech with the corresponding movements. In eurythmy we bring back what attended the vowels and consonants as movements and thus

13

bring the body into movement again. Now we must realize that when we pronounce vowels we omit the movement and make the vowel inward, that previously joined in the outward movement to an extent. We take something away from it on its path to the interior. We take the movement away. Thus we restore to the vowel in outer movement what we have taken away from it on its inward-going path. In the case of the vowel, matters are such that the outward movement is of exceptional importance in the search for the transferal of the effect of the vowel, eurythmically expressed, onto the whole man. That is what we must take into account here.

In speaking of vowels today, we will speak purely of the meaning of that which is eurythmically vocalized in movement. Here it is very important that one develops a feeling for what flows into the movement. That one develops a perceptive consciousness which tells one whether that which is happening in the respective human limb is a stretching, a rounding, or such. One must decidedly acquire a specific consciousness for this. In what pertains to vowels it is extremely important that one feels the movement made or the position taken up. That is what is important. Starting from here, we will transpose each of the vowels from the eurythmic into the therapeutic.

Practically demonstrated (Mrs. Baumann): a distinct "I" made by stretching both arms. This stretching should be carried out in such a way that one then returns (to the rest position; the ed.) and performs the same movement somewhat lower, returns again, and does it with both (arms) horizontal. Now we go back and, if you had the right forward at first, now, as you go lower, you must take the right to the back, and now to the front, now a bit back again, and then somewhat deeper. Now I don't want to trouble you further with that, but if one wanted to carry it out, one could make it more complicated by taking more positions; one would then start with the "I", return, do it a little further on, go back, a bit further on, and so forth, so that one has as many "I"-positions as possible, carried out from above to below, always returning (to the rest position; the ed.). When these movements are performed, they are an expression for the human being as a person. The entire individual person is thereby expressed.

Now we could notice for example that some child, for that matter a grown up person, cannot express himself properly as a person. He is somehow inhibited in the expression of himself as a complete individuality. He might be a dreamer in a certain sense or something similar. Or, if we think of a physical abnormality — in the case of a child, for example, that he doesn't learn to walk properly, he walks clumsily — or if in the case of an adult we notice that it would be desirable for hygienic or therapeutic reasons that the person learn to walk better, this particular exercise would be very good for this. When grown-ups step out too little in their stride, when they don't reach out properly with their steps, it always means that the circulation suffers under it. The circulation of the blood suffers under an insufficiently outreaching gait. So when people walk in this way (lightly tripping; the ed.), that has a consequence that the circulation becomes in some fashion slower than it should be in that person. Then one must attempt to have this person learn to step out again, and by having him do this exercise, one will be certain to attain one's goal. Then the person will have greater and more penetrating results in learning to walk properly. Thus one can say that in essence this modified "I"-exercise furthers those people who — I will express it somewhat radically — cannot walk properly. It can be summed up approximately so: for people who cannot walk properly.

You can extend the exercise further, and, with the addition of a sort of resumée of what Mrs. Baumann has done, it will be that much more effective. Now try to do the whole exercise without bringing the arms back (to the rest position; the ed.) so that you reach the last position only by turning:

15

turning in a plane, quick, quicker and quicker. The "I"-exercise as it was first demonstrated and described can be intensified in this way and will benefit those people who cannot walk properly. It will then be extraordinarily easy to bring them to walk properly. One can admonish them to walk properly and their efforts to walk in a different manner will bring suitable results as well.

Now Mrs. Baumann will demonstrate an "U"-exercise for us. The arms quite high up, and back to the starting position, now a bit lower, back again, a little lower, now horizontal, back again, now below, back again, and again below; that is the principle of it. And now do it straightaway so that you start above maintaining the "U" as you move downwards; and now do it increasingly quickly so that at last you reach quite a speed.

Please keep this in mind as the manner in which to execute the "U"-exercise. If I were to summarize again in the same fashion as earlier, I would call this the movement for children or adults who cannot stand. In the case of "I" we had those who cannot walk, with "U", we have those who cannot stand.

Now not being able to stand is to have weak feet and to become very easily tired when standing. It would also mean, for example, that one could not stand long enough on tiptoe properly, or that one could not stand on one's heels long enough without immediately becoming clumsy. Standing on tiptoe or on the heels are no eurythmic exercises, but they should be practised by people who have weak legs, who tire easily while standing or who can't stand properly at all. To be unable to stand properly is to be easily tired in walking as well. That is a technical difference: to walk awkwardly and to tire in walking are two different things. When the person is tired by walking, one has to do with the "U"-exercise. When the person walks clumsily or when as a result of his whole constitution it would be desirable for him to learn to step out with his feet, that can be technically expressed as

16

being unable to walk. However, to be tired by walking would be technically expressed as not being able to stand. And for such people the "U"-exercise is especially appropriate. This is interrelated with matters with which we must deal once we have come a bit further.

Now please do the "O"-movement: quite high up and back (to the rest position; the ed.) and now somewhat lower, back again, lower still, and so on. Now do it so that you make the "O"-movement above; feel distinctly the rounding of the arms within the movement as you glide down. When you glide down with the "O"-movement it must remain an "O". Now increasingly faster.

You would see this exercise complete in its most brilliant application if you had here in front of you a really corpulent person. If a child or grown-up becomes unnaturally fat, then this is the exercise to be applied. By making the "O" so often and by extending it to this barrel-shaped body at the end — then it is really a barrel that one describes outside oneself — that which forms the opposite pole to those dynamic tendencies at work in making a person obese is in fact carried out. One can apply it very well hygienically and therapeutically, and you will be convinced that a tendency to become thinner actually appears when you have such people carry out this movement, especially when they practise other things as well which we have as yet to discuss. But at the same time it is of special significance in this exercise that you have the person practise only so long as he can without sweating heavily and becoming too warm. If one wishes to attain the desired effect, one must try to conduct the exercise so that the person can always rest in between.

Now Mrs. Baumann will make an "E"-movement, quite high above. It is a proper "E"-movement only when this hand lies on the other so that they touch. Now return (to the rest position; the ed.), then somewhat lower, the right hand over the left arm, and then, so that it is really effective, we will do it so that it lies increasingly further back and now again from above to below; then the "E" must be done so that it penetrates thoroughly. And now, in bringing it down, you must move (the crossing) further back, so far that you split the shoulder seam at the back. Now this is the exercise that will be especially advantageous for weaklings, that is to say, for thin people rather than fat people, for those people in whom the weakness comes distinctly from within, but is organically conditioned. It must be organically caused.

Another exercise which can be considered parallel to this should be applied with some caution as it affects the soul more closely. It is the following: make an "E" to the rear as well as you can and as far up as you can. That really hurts. It is a movement that is in itself a bit painful and that is indeed the purpose. It should be practised with those children or adults in whom there are psychological grounds for becoming thin, such as being worn down and so on. Since one must in principle be careful in approaching from the outside with healing by such spiritual means, this too must of course be applied with caution. That means that one must inspire a child who has failed or who shows signs of depression so that he takes heart when one will have him do these exercises. If one concerns oneself with the child otherwise by comforting him and caring for his soul, then one can have him do these exercises as well.

You can see that in the case of all these things it is to a degree a matter of extending what comes to expression in artistic eurythmy in a certain manner. This is especially true in respect to the vowels.

Now it is very important that we make the following clear to ourselves. You know that the vowel element can be developed in this fashion, and that it is in essence the expression of the inward. One must only grasp through feeling and contemplation that which takes place. One must bear in mind that the person concerned, the person who carries out these things in order to be healed, must feel them; in "E" he feels that one arm covers the other. In the case of "O" however,

18

something more comes into consideration. In "O" one should feel not only the closing of the circle, but the bending as well. One should feel that one is building a circle. One should feel the circle that runs through it. And in order to make the "O" particularly effective one should make the person doing it aware as well that he should feel as though he himself or someone else were to draw a line along his breastbone, thus by means of feeling, closing the whole to the rear in spirit; as if one were to experience something like having a line drawn on the breastbone by oneself or someone else.

Now we want to make an "A": we return (to the rest position; the ed.), now we make an "A" somewhat lower, return again, make an "A" horizontally, back, make an "A" somewhat lowered, back, an "A" very deep, back, then to the rear; that you need to do only once, but return first (to the rest positon; the ed.). And now make the "A" above and without changing the angle bring it down, and, again without the feeling that you change the angle, to the back.

This exercise can be really effective only if one has it done frequently. And when one has it repeated frequently, it is the exercise to be used with people who are greedy, in whom the animal nature comes particularly strongly to the fore. So if you have in school a child who is in every way a proper little animal, and in whom the condition has an organic cause, when you have him do this exercise, you will see that it has for him a very particular significance.

In the case of these exercises you can observe once again that if they are to be introduced into the school it will be necessary to organize the children into groups especially for them. You will soon become convinced that the children do these exercises much less gladly than the other eurythmic exercises. While they are eager to do the others, one will most likely have to persuade them to do these, as they will react at first as children often react to taking medicine: with resistance. They won't be particularly happy about it, but that is of no especial harm in the exercises having to do with "O", "U",

"E", and "A"; in the case of "I" it is somewhat harmful when the child doesn't enjoy it. One must try to reach the stage where the children delight in the "I"-exercise as we have done it. In the case of the others, "U", "O", "E", and "A", it is not especially damaging if they carry out the exercise on authority, and knowing that it is their duty to do it. With "I" it is important that the children have pleasure in doing it as it affects the whole individual, as I have said already.

You will profit further by coming to terms with the following: the "I" reveals man as a person, the "U" reveals man as man, the "O" reveals man as soul, the "E" fixes the ego in the etheric body, it permeates the etheric body, strongly with the ego. And the "A" counteracts the animal nature in man.

Now we will follow the various workings further. If you have a person with irregular breathing, who is in some fashion burdened down by his breathing and such like, you will be able to bring this person to normal breathing by applying the vowels. You will be able to achieve in particular the distinct articulation of the consonants by means of these exercises, as that is greatly facilitated through the practice of the vowels. When you notice that certain children cannot manage to form certain consonants with the lips or the tongue — for the palatal sounds (Gaumenlaute) it is less applicable, although for the labial and lingual sounds exceptionally good — it will be of great help to the children with difficulties in this respect, when one tries to have them do such exercises as early as possible.

You will also notice that when people tend to chronic headaches, to migrane-like conditions, these can be appreciably alleviated through the practice of the vowels. So in the cases of chronic headaches and chronic migrane symptoms, as well as when people are foggy-headed, these things will be particularly applicable. Similarly, if you employ the exercises which we have done today for children who cannot pay attention, who are sleepy, you will awaken them in a certain sense to a state of awareness. That is a hygienic-didactic angle of a certain significance. It will be observed that sleepy-headed adults can definitely be awakened in this way as well. And then one will notice that when a person's digestion is too weak or too slow, that by means of these exercises this slow digestion and all that is known to be connected with it, can be changed for the better.

In certain forms of hygienic eurythmy it would be good to have the movements — which are carried out with the arms only in artistic eurythmy — done with the legs as well where possible, only somewhat less forcefully, as I am about to describe. Now you will ask how one can make an "I", for example, with the legs? It's very easy. One must only stretch out the leg and feel the stretching in it. The "U" would be simply to stand with full awareness on both legs, so that one has a distinct stretching feeling in both. "O" with legs must be learned, however. One should really accustom the people with whom one finds it necessary to do the "O"-exercise in the manner that I have described, to do the "O" with the legs as well. That consists in pointing the toes somewhat, but only very slightly, to the outside and then trying to stand in this manner and hold one's position. One must thereby stand on tiptoe, however, and bend outward, remain so standing a moment and then return to the normal position; then build it up again and so on.

It is necessary to take into account the relationship existing between the possibilities of organically determined inner movement in the middle man and the lower man. This is such that movement done for the lower man should be carried out at only one-third the strength. Thus when you have someone carry out the "O" movement as we have seen it, you must have the feeling that what is done later for the legs and feet requires only one-third of the time and thus only a third of the energy expended. It will be especially effective, however, when you place this in the middle, so that you have, let us

21

say, A and then A again, with B, the foot movement, in the middle (see the table); it will be particularly effective to have them together.

one-third	one-third	one-third
A	B	A
Arm	Foot	Arm

It will also be especially effective to do the same in connection with the "E"-exercise for the feet, by really crossing the feet.

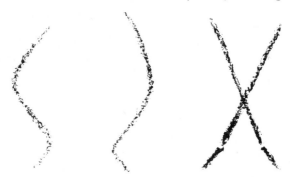

But one must stand on tiptoe and lay one leg over the other so that they touch. Again, one-third, and placed, if possible, in the middle. That is something which it would be particularly good to have done by children, and by adults as well, who are weaklings. They will naturally be hardly capable of doing it, but that is exactly why they must learn to do it. In precisely these matters one sees that that which it is most important for various people to learn is that which they are most incapable of doing. They must learn it because it is necessary to the recovery of their health.

"A" (with the legs; the ed.) is also necessary; I have already demonstrated it to you yesterday. It consists in assuming this spread position while standing insofar as it is possible on tiptoe. That should also be introduced into the A-movement and it will be particularly effective there.

Now one can also intensify all the exercises that we have just described by carrying them out in walking. And you will achieve a great deal for a weak child, for example, when you teach him to do the "E"-motion as we have just done it in walking; he should walk in such a manner that he always touches each leg alternately. In taking a step forward he crosses over first with one leg, then with the other, so that he always crosses one leg over the other, so that he places one leg at the back and touches it with the other in front. Naturally he won't move ahead very well, but it is good to have this movement carried out while walking. You will say that complicated movements appear as a result; but it is good when complicated movements appear.

Now I want to bring it to your attention that what we have said about the vowel element should be sharply distinguished to begin with from what we will practice tomorrow in respect to the consonants. The consonantal element is such that it generally expresses the external, as we have already said. In speech as well the consonant is so formed that a reconstruction, an imitation of the outer form comes into being through the formative motions of lips and tongue. Now the consonants have, as we will see tomorrow, very special sorts of movements and it lies within these forms of movement to make the consonant inward again in a certain manner by giving it eurythmic form. It is internalized. That which it loses in the outward-going path of speech is restored to it. And, whether one is contemplating them in eurythmy as art or performing them for personal reasons, in the case of consonants it is particularly important to have, not a feeling in the way one does with a vowel, a feeling of stretching, of bending, or of widening and so on, but to imagine oneself simultaneously in the form that one carries out while making the consonants, as though one were to observe oneself.

Here you can see most clearly that one must admonish the artistic eurythmists not to mix the two things; the artistic eurythmists would not do well to observe themselves constantly as they would rob themselves of their ability to work unselfconsciously. On the contrary, when you have a child or

23

a grown-up carry out something having to do with consonants, it is important that they photograph themselves inwardly in their thought as it were; then in this inward photographing of oneself lies that which is effective; the person must really see himself inwardly in the position that he is carrying out and it must be performed in such a manner that the person has an inner picture of what he does.

If you would be so good (Miss Wolfram) as to show us an "M" as a consonant, first with the right hand, now with the left, but taking it backwards, now taking the right hand back, and "M" with the left hand and now with both hands, that can be multiplied in various ways, of course. Now an "M" — we will start with this example; to begin with, what is it as speech? In speech "M" is an extraordinarily important sound. You will experience its importance in speech, and in speech physiology as well, if you contrast it with the "S". Perhaps Mrs. Baumann will make a graceful "S" for us now, right, left, and now with both hands.

Now to begin with it appears that you have the feeling, or should have the feeling when the "S" is done that you encounter something within you — it is the etheric body namely (at this point Dr. Steiner made the corresponding movement; the ed.); so that you have a snake-like line. This serpentine may approach a straight line in the case of a

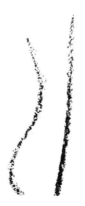

particularly sharply pronounced "S" and can even be represented as a straight line. By contrast, when you look at the "M" that was just performed, you should have the feeling — even when the organic form is carried out inwardly — that it is really not the same thing. And so the "M" is that which counters the "S"-direction when laid against it and that is in essence the great polarity between an "S" and an "M";

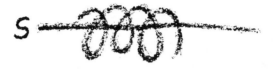

they are two polar sounds. "S" is the truly Ahrimanic sound, if I may speak anthroposophically, and the "M" is that which mitigates the properties of the Ahrimanic, makes it mild; if I may express it so, it takes its Ahrimanic strength from it. So when we have a combination of sounds directly including "S" and "M", for example "Samen" (seed) or "Summe" (sum), we have in this combination of sounds first the strong Ahrimanic being in "S", whose sting is then taken from it by the "M".

Perhaps you will make a "H" for us (Miss Wolfram). When you really look at the "H", when you feel yourself really within this "H", then, you will say to yourself: there is something in this "H" which reveals itself as unequivocally Luciferic. It is the Luciferic in the "H", then, which comes to expression here. And now try to observe yourself — here the feeling is less important than the contemplation of it — try to observe yourself, when Mrs. Baumann does it for us now, how it is when one does the "H" and allows it to go over immediately into an "M". Make the "H" first and let it carry over by and by into an "M". Now take a look at it. In this movement you have the whole perception of the mitigation of the Luciferic, of its sting being taken from it, brought to expression. The movement is truly as if one would arrest Lucifer. And, one can also hear it if you simply think about it — today's civilized man can actually no longer reflect properly on these things. If someone wants to agree to something Luciferic, but immediately diminishes the actual Luciferic element, the eagerness of his assent, then he says, "Hm, hm". There you have the "H" and the "M" placed really very close to one another and you have the whole charm of the diminished Luciferic directly within it.

From this you can see that as soon as one turns to the consonantal element, one must immediately turn to the observation of the form as well. That is the essential thing and tomorrow we will speak about it further.

LECTURE 3

Dornach, April 14, 1921

In order to proceed in an appropriate manner, we will prepare the grounds today for certain matters to be deepened physiologically and psychologically tomorrow, considering the forms which consonants take in eurythmic movement. In what has been developed as the form involved in consonantal movement consideration has been truly given to everything which must be taken into account when man attempts to penetrate into the outer world through speech. The person who sets himself the task of observing speech will see that man's confrontation with the outer world must consist on the one hand of living into the world vigorously; of making himself selfless and living out into the world. In the vowels he comes to himself; in the vowels he goes within and unfolds his activity there. In the consonants he becomes in a way one with the outer world although to varying degrees. These varying degrees of unification with the world are manifest in certain practices within language as well. In the development of the consonantal element in eurythmy, particularly in reference to the sensible-supersensible observation of which I so often speak in introducing eurythmy performances, — it is necessary to take into consideration whether the human being objectifies himself. To discover whether man extroverts himself completely in order to grasp the spiritual element in the things outside him in a spoken sound, or if, despite this objectification of himself, he remains more within and does not go completely out of himself but instead reproduces the external within himself. That is a major distinction, by reason of which I must ask Mrs. Baumann to be so good and show us first of all the movement for "H". Now please disregard this H-movement altogether and Mrs. Baumann will demonstrate the F-movement. And now keep an eye on what you can observe here in these two different movements. You can observe what is present by virtue of the human instinct in the attempt to enunciate the sound in question. Consider the pronunciation of H: actually you say H-a, you follow up with a vowel. It is impossible to sound a consonant without it being tinged by a vowel, you follow it up with an "A". The pure consonant is vocalized, combined with a vowel. If you consider the "F" you will find that man's linguistic instinct places an "E" in front of it: e-F. Here the opposite occurs: an E is set before it.

Through the foregoing you will perceive that when man utters an "H" he makes a greater effort to uncover through speech the spiritual in the external object; when he utters an "F" his effort is directed more towards re-experiencing the spiritual within himself. Therefore the manner in which the consonant arises is entirely different, according to whether the vowel tinges the consonant from the front or from the back, if I may use this manner of expression in respect to the nature of consonantal articulation. This you will find conveyed in the form you have observed.

Perhaps Miss Wolfram will do the "H" once again. H: here you have an energetic unfolding in the outer world, one doesn't wish to remain in oneself, one wants to go out and live in the external. F: you see the decided effort to avoid entering into the outer world too sharply, to remain in the inner.

Now when one takes this into consideration, one can carry on from here to form a mental picture of various matters which, although they must become part of eurythmy, were, to begin with, unnecessary as far as we have been concerned with eurythmy as art, but which will become necessary the more this art is extended to other languages. The moment one says not "ef" but "fi", in that moment it is a different matter; in that moment one attempts to embrace the external with the sound as well. This is indicative of an important historical fact: In ancient Greece people attempted to grasp the external even in those things in respect to which modern man has become inward. You see how one can follow into the outermost fringes of man's experience what I have expressed for example, in *The Riddles of Philosophy*:* this going out and taking hold in the external world of what man today already experiences entirely inwardly in his ego. The reason why spiritual science is not accepted on the grounds of such things is solely that the people of our civilization are in general too lazy. They have to take too many things into account in order to come to the truth, and they want to make it easier for themselves. But that just won't do. They want to make *everything* easier for themselves; and that won't do.

That, for the present, in respect to one element which flowed into the formation of the consonants. If we want to understand the formation of consonants in the field of eurythmy, then we should consider a second element which I believe people pay less attention to nowadays in teaching, even in physiology, speech physiology, than the third element which we will come to in a moment. In order to form an impression, I will ask you to compare once again. Here it is important that one form a contemplative picture. Naturally, one cannot penetrate to the very end of that which one has in such a picture, to the concept.

Perhaps Mrs. Baumann will be so good and make the H again, and once the tone has faded away, Mrs. Baumann will make a D for us. One must pay attention in this case to the following: When you contemplate the H, you will find the movement for it deviates greatly to begin with from what takes place in speaking it; since — in respect to the characteristic of which I am thinking at the moment — the

* Published by the Anthroposophic Press, Inc., New York, 1973.

eurythmic element must be polar to the actual process in speech. You know that the speech process as I presented it the day before yesterday is a reflecting back from the larynx. The eurythmic process must express this outwardly. It expresses it in movement. In certain instances one must go over to the exactly opposite pole. This is particularly characteristic of H and D; in the case of other consonants this element must be toned down. Now, what sort of a sound is H? H is esentially a breath sound. The H is actually brought into being through blowing. In the case of H you have a decided shoving thrust* in eurythmy where you have to blow. When you utter "D" you have this thrusting effect* in the pronunciation. We must polarize this by transforming it into the characteristic movement that was present in D. Thus the thrusting quality of speech is lamed when one conveys the sound through movement.

So you see that precisely this characteristic must be taken into particular account, when one has either a breath sound or a plosive sound. Now sounds are not only either breath or plosive sounds. But by what reason are they one or the other? You see, when one has a decided breath sound, one expresses by means of the blowing the fact that one really wants to go out of oneself; in the thrusting,* that this going out of oneself is difficult, that one would like to remain within. For this reason the eurythmic transposition of the sound must take place in the manner you have seen.

Now one also has sounds that carefully connect the inward with the outward; sounds that are actually physiologically so constituted that with them one states that one is bringing to a standstill, arresting, that in which one would like to be active in such a manner that the inward would immediately become outward, where one would enter into the movement immediately with the whole human being. This is decidedly evident in only one sound in our language: the R, which is,

* stossige wirkung

30

however, for this reason the most inclusive sound; one would like to run after the speech organism with every limb, as I would like to express it, when one says R. Actually with R one strives to bring this pursuit to rest. The lips want to follow when they pronounce the labial R, and bring this running-after to a halt, the tongue wants to follow when it speaks the lingual R, and finally the palate wants to follow when the palatal R sounds. These three R's are distinctly different from one another, but are nevertheless one; in eurythmy they are expressed thus (Mrs. Baumann: R). The bringing-in-swing of what one usually brings to a standstill is expressed. Thus it is precisely the running after the movement of the sound that comes to expression in the R. And when one wants to bring the other element to expression, one can express the labial R by carrying the movement further downwards; the lingual R can be made more in the horizontal and the palatal R rather more upwards. By this means one can modify the R-sound in the eurythmic movement. But you see that the form is determined by leaving the vibration of the R in the background and bringing the "running-after" to expression.

A similar sound where one has, not a vibrating, but a sort of wave in the movement is the L (Miss Wolfram: L). You see that there is something of the same movement in it as in the R; but the running-after is mild and comes to rest. It is a wave rather than a vibration that comes to expression.

That is what is connected innerly, physiologically, with the shading through the vowel element of the consonantal sound, and with the shading through feeling, which already leads to a greater extent into the physical. One arrives at the outermost division of the sounds by considering the organs; if we compare once again the respective movements we will arrive at the most extreme, the most external principles of division through our contemplative picture. (Mrs. Baumann: B) That is a B, and now we will continue directly perhaps with a T. (Mrs. Baumann: T). Now you can see from the

31

position — which as the third element must be taken into account and which makes itself quite apparent to the sensible-supersensible contemplation — that in the case of B we have to do with a labial sound and in the case of T with a dental sound. (Miss Wolfram: K) K: here one starts with the position and the essential lies in the movement. Here we have to do with a palatal sound which in its pronounciation, in the tone in which it is spoken is the quietest, but which is transformed in movement into its polar opposite when performed outwardly in eurythmy. The consonants overlap in respect to their characteristics; one division extends into another. The following may serve as an aid.

Take the labial sounds — I'll write out only the most distinctive of them: V, B, P, F, M. You can determine to what extent the vowel colouring is involved by pronouncing the sounds; I don't need to indicate that. Let us take the dental sounds D, T, S, Sh, L, the English Th, and N. And now the palatal sounds: G, K, Ch, and the French Ng, more or less. We will have to write the R in everywhere, since it has its nuances everywhere:

Labial sounds:	V, B, P, F, M	R
Dental sounds:	D, T, S, Sh, L, (Th), N	R
Palatal sounds:	G, K, Ch, Ng	R

Considering the process of division from the other point of view now, I will underline with white where we have to do with a definite breath sound: V, F, S, Sh and Ch as well, more or less. These would be the decided breath sounds. I will underline in red where we have to do with what are clearly plosive sounds: B, P, M, D, T, N, and then perhaps G and K. The vibratory sound is R. We have to do with a distinct undulent sound — which, because of the soft transformation in the movement, must be in a sense of an inward character — fundamentally only in the case of L.

These three organizational principles — the vowel colouring, the blowing, thrusting, vibrating and undulating, and all that which has to do with the external division (into dental, labial and palatal sounds; the ed.) – all this comes to expression in the forms given for eurythmy. It must be clear to you, of course, to what degree these principles of division affect each other, however. When we have to do with L, for example, we have to do with a distinct dental sound which must have all the characteristics of a dental sound, and then we have to do with a gliding sound, with an undulant sound, which must have the characteristics of a wave. Apart from that, it has a strong connection to the inward. We have to do with a colouring from within outwards, at least in our language. We don't say "le", but "el"; here we have the transition from older forms in which people reached yearningly into the exterior world and where as a result a word was used in order to express such an event, in order to bring this going over into the external to proper expression. Thus in each of the letters we have to do with a likeness of that which is taking place inwardly.

Before we consider the consonants individually, let us contemplate the following. Yesterday we were able to show that A – which we also studied in its metamorphosis – has to do with all those forces in man that make him greedy, which organize him according to animal nature: the A in fact lies nearest to the animal nature in man, and in a certain sense one can say that when the A is pronounced it sounds out of the animality of man. And certainly as spiritual investigation confirms A is the sound which was the very earliest to appear in the course of both the phylogenetic evolution as well as the ontogenetic evolution of man. In ontogenetic evolution it is somewhat hidden of course; there is a false evolution as well, as you know. The A was the first sound to appear in the evolution of mankind, however, resounding to begin with entirely out of the animal nature. And when we tend towards A with the consonants, we are still calling on what are animal forces in man. As you could see yesterday, the whole sound is actually formed accordingly. If we use the sound therapeutically in the manner in which it presented itself to our souls yesterday we can combat that which makes children, and grown-ups too, into smaller and larger animals. With such exercises we can have very respectable results in the de-animalization of man.

And now let us go on to the sound U, for example. We said yesterday that this is the sound we use therapeutically when a person cannot stand. You saw that yesterday. It is the sound which in a certain respect expresses its physiologic-pathologic connection already in the manner in which it is formed in speech. The U is spoken with the mouth and the openings between the teeth constricted to the greatest degree and with the lips somewhat extended, in such a way, however, that the mouth opening is narrowed and the lips can vibrate. You can see that in speaking one seeks an essentially outward movement with the U. In the pronounciation of U the attempt to characterize something moving predominates. Thus with the eurythmic U the physiologic opposite occurs: the ability to hold one's stand is called forth. This is present in the U in artistic eurythmy as well, at least as a suggestion.

If you now take a look at the other vowels you will find a progressive internalization. In the case of the O you have the lips pushed together towards the front and the opening of the mouth reduced in size — there is at least an attempt to reduce the size. This is transformed into the polar opposite in the encompassing gesture of the O-movement in eurythmy. Precisely in such things the natural connections are to be perceived. In the manner in which O is employed in speech certain forces are present. And in languages in which O predominates one will find that the people have the greatest propensity to become obese. That may really be taken as a guideline for the study of the physiologic processes connected with speech. If one were to develop a language consisting principally of modifications of O, where people had to carry out the characteristic mouth and lip formation of the O continuously, they would all become pot-bellied. If with the O, on the one hand, one has this propensity to become big-bellied, as I would like to call it, it is easy to understand why when reversed the O represents on the other hand that which combats this obesity when it is carried out eurythmically and in the metamorphosis demonstrated yesterday.

The state of affairs is different with E, for example. A language that is rich in E will engender skinny people, weaklings. And that is related to what I said yesterday about the treatment of thin people, and thus of weaklings, in relation to the significance of E. You will remember that I said that in the case of weaklings particularly the E-movement with its given modification is to be applied.

Now in respect to all these matters it is necessary to take one thing into account, however: if one considers the forms outwardly one does not come to the truth of the matter; one must grasp them inwardly in the process of their becoming. One must concentrate less on what comes to outward expression and more on the tendency involved. The tendency to become fat can be combated by means of the O and the tendency to remain thin by the E. Attention must be drawn to these matters because when eurythmy is used for therapeutic purposes, it is necessary to take the forces that are present in the upper man and tend to a widening, and the forces present in the lower man tending to the linear, more into consideration. Thus I must say that when man utters the O he actually broadens the living element.

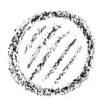

You see, when I draw it roughly, the head of man is in a way a sphere and spiritual-scientifically it is a proper reproduction of the earth sphere. It is a copy of all those forces that are centralized in the sphere of the earth and it is developed by that which lies in the forces of the moon. This latter builds it up in such a manner that it becomes a sort of earth-sphere. Of course, this is all actually connected with cosmology, cosmogeny. As the earth-phase proceeded out of the moon-phase, so out of the forces that are so powerfully at work in building up the human head — which of itself, of course, intends to become a sphere and is modified only by the breast and the other part of the body being attached to it and altering the spherical form — so out of the moon-building forces the head is formed. If it were left to itself the head would become a proper sphere. That is not the case because the other two parts of the human organism are connected with the head and influence its shape.

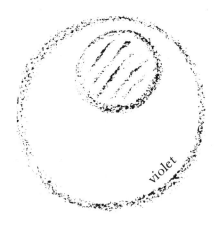

When one pronounces the O one tries to bring that which finds its expression in the spherical form of the head to expression in the entire etheric head. One makes the effort to form a second head for oneself (see the violet in the drawing) and one can really say that in uttering the O man puffs himself up like his head — he puffs himself up, he blows himself out and awakens thereby the forces that give him at the other pole the tendency to become fat. These things can really be taken pictorially as well. His inflating of his own head gives him the tendency to become fat. When one wants to counteract this tendency to become, etherically-speaking, a fat-head — not really a fat-head, but etherically a fat head — to become a big head, then one must attempt to round it off from the other side, to take it back into oneself. And that is the protest of the fathead. Therefore an O is formed at the opposite pole. All the individual sounds have a nuance of feeling, namely, which is deeply established in the organism, because it lies in the unconscious; hence the import of the inner being of the sound. For the person who looks at the matter in a supersensible manner the frog who would like to blow himself up into an ox, you see, is the one from whom a cannon-like O tone would continuously proceed if he were able to fulfill his intention. That is the peculiarity of it — one must explain by means of such things if one wishes to understand these matters inwardly.

With the E it is distinctly the reverse. In E one wants to take hold of oneself inwardly, wants to contract together inwardly. For that reason there is the touching of oneself in the eurythmy, this becoming aware of oneself: you become aware of yourself, simply, when you place the right arm upon the left, just as when you feel an object outside yourself, when you take a hold of it, you become aware of yourself. It would be even more clearly expressed if you simply grasped the right arm with the left hand — in art only an indication of all these things can be given — when you grasp the right arm with the left hand you are feeling yourself. This contacting oneself has come to expression especially in the eurythmic E. And this touching oneself is carried out throughout the whole human organism. You can study this touching of oneself simply by studying the relationship of the nerve process in the human back, those that ordinary physiology mistakenly call the motory nerves and those that are called sensory.

Here where the motor nerve, which is basically a sensory nerve too, comes together with the sensory nerve, a similar sort of clasping occurs. The fact is that the nerve-strands on the human back continually form an E. In this forming of the E lies the way in which man's inward perception of himself which is factually differentiated, in the brain, comes into being. Yesterday we attempted to reproduce this E-building which actually takes place in a plane; you will find that what we attempted to reproduce shows through the outward movement and the position of the movement how this inward E-making in man sums itself up into the vertical. As the head puffs itself out and wants to become a horn-blowing cherub, this E-process, this pulling-oneself-together-in-points, sums itself up in the vertical, in the upright line. It is a continuous and successive fastening together of E's which stand one above another; that expresses clearly what one observes taking place in weaklings. They have the tendency to continuously stretch their etheric bodies. They want to extend the etheric body rather than to pull it together into a point, which would be the real antithesis to the activity of the head. That is not the case however: they try to stretch the etheric body thereby making a repetition of the point. And this extension which makes its appearance in people who are becoming weak — not the extension in the physical, but in the etheric body — will be counteracted by shaping that E of which we spoke yesterday.

So I believe you will see now how there is an inward connection between the eurythmic element involved and the human formative tendencies, how what is present in him as formative tendencies has been drawn out of the human being. The fact is that these formative tendencies which express themselves first in growth, in the forming of man, in his configuration, become specialized and localized once again in the development of the speech organism, this special organism. There these formative tendencies — which are otherwise spread out over the entire person — are to an extent accumulated. In developing eurythmy we turn and go back again. We proceed from the localized tendency to the whole

38

man, thus placing in opposition to the specialization of the human organization in the speech organism another specialization, the specialization in the will-organism. The whole human being is indeed an expression of his volitional nature insofar as he is metabolic and limb organism throughout. One can move this or that part of the head too, and therefore the head is also in a certain sense limb-organism. That can be demonstrated by those people who are capable in this respect of a bit more than others. People who can wiggle their ears and so on, they can show very clearly how the principle of movement of the limbs, how the limb-nature extends into the organization of the head. The whole human being is in this respect an expression of the volitional. When we go on to eurythmy we express that once again. Before we proceed to working out the sounds particularly, to the special manner of forming them and further to the combinations of sounds tomorrow, I would like to speak in closing of something historical.

The movement of the will and the movement of the intellect, you see, constitute two sorts of evolution of power which proceed in man at different velocities. Man's intellect develops quickly in our age, volition slowly, so that as part of the whole evolution of mankind we have already surpassed our will with our intellect. In our civilization it is generally manifest that the evolution of the intellect has overtaken the evolution of the will. The people of today are intensely intellectual, which precisely does not imply that they can do much with their intellect; they are strongly intellectual, but they hardly know what to do with their intellect; for that reason they know so little intellectually. But what they do know intellectually they treat in such a manner as though within it they could function with a certain certainty. Will develops slowly. And to practise eurythmy is, apart from everything else, an attempt to bring the will back into the whole evolution of mankind again. If eurythmy is to appear as a therapy the following must be pointed out: It must be said that the over-development of the intellect expresses

39

itself particularly in the organic side effects of the evolution of speech as well. Our speech development today in our modern civilization is actually already something which is becoming inhuman through its superhuman qualities insofar as we learn languages today in such a manner that we have so little living feeling left for what lies in the words. The words are actually only signs. What sort of feeling do people still have for that which lies in words? I would like to know how many people go through the world and become aware in the course of learning the German language for example, that the rounded form which I have just drawn is expressed in the word "Kopf" (Head), which has a connection with "Kohl" (cabbage), and for which reason one also says "Kohlkopf" (cabbagehead), which is actually only a repetition; the rounding is metamorphosed according to the situation. That is what is expressed here. In the Romance languages, "testa, testieren", is expressed more what comes from within, the working of the soul through the head. People have no more feeling for the distinctions within language; language has become abstract. When you walk, you walk with you feet. Why do we say "Füsse" (feet)? You see, that is a metamorphosis of the word "Furche" (furrow) which came about because it was seen that one traces something like a furrow when one walks. The pictorial element in language has been completely lost; if one wishes to bring this pictorial element back into language, then one must turn to eurythmy.

Every word that is experienced unpictorially is actually an inward cause of illness; I am speaking in coarse words now — but then we have only coarse words — of something which expresses itself in the finer human organism. Civilized mankind suffers chronically today from the effects which learning to speak abstractly, which the failure to experience words pictorially, has upon it. The results are so far-reaching that the accompanying organic side effects express themselves as a very strong tendency towards irregularities in the rhythmic system and a refusal to function of the metabolic

40

system in those people who have made their language abstract. However, we can actually do something about what is being spoilt in man today through language, which he acquires of course in early childhood, and which, if it is acquired in an unpictorial way, really produces conditions leading later on to all kinds of illnesses. We can actually do something about overcoming this with the help of therapeutic eurythmy. Thus curative eurythmy may be introduced in a thoroughly organic manner into the course of therapy as a whole.

It is truly so: the person who understands that developing oneself spiritually has always something to do with becoming ill — we must take becoming ill in the course of spiritual development into the bargain — must also taken into consideration that one can fight, not alone through outward physical studies, but also by outward means, this process of becoming ill which is due to our civilization. We put soul and spirit into the movements of eurythmy and combat thereby what, on the other side, soul and spirit do themselves, though often in earliest childhood, in such a manner that the effect of their activity when it develops in later life must be felt to be the cause of illness.

LECTURE 4

Dornach, April 15, 1921

As we have seen the vowels in eurythmy always work more or less directly on the rhythmic organism. With the consonantal eurythmic movements the case is that, although the rhythmic organism is, of course, also affected, this is accomplished by way of the limb-metabolic system. Naturally the first thing we must do today is simply to take a look at the details; here one can only arrive at a contemplative picture of what is involved when one can enter into the details. We will now go through the most important consonantal movements in eurythmy. Perhaps you would make a B for us, Miss Wolfram; and now this B in walking as well. Try to walk in such a manner, however, that one leg imitates the motion of the arm while moving; but repeat the B. Now imagine that done more and more quickly and repeated to begin with, let us say for four to five minutes. Perhaps Mrs. Baumann will now do the P for us in the same manner. The difference is not very great. Now you must attempt to do this with the legs as well. That brings about a complicated leg movement which is very similar to the movements of tone eurythmy. That must now be repeated frequently and in series by the person with whom one hopes to accomplish something by means of the P.

Now all of the movements that are connected with the eurythmic consonants have to do with that in the process of digestion which lies on the far side of the activity of the stomach and intestine. We will now ignore the actual intestinal space through which the food passes. When we consider the outer wall of the intestine, however, where the chyme passes

42

through the intestinal villi and so on and then into the blood and the lymph — thus from the other side of that comprised in the first digestive activity — movement such as we have just made work back on the inward digestion, on all that which is digestive activity in the blood vessels, and moreover on what is digestive activity in the kidneys. Thus if you should be concerned with regulating the activity of the kidneys, you should have such movements carried out. Precisely the movements which we have just done, B and P, are those which work pre-eminently in the regulation of renal activity, for example in regulating the elimination of urine. These connections are certainly extraordinarily interesting for someone who remembers how the whole circulatory being of man is related to language, and how a connection thus arises between that which pushes itself into the circulatory system from the metabolic system and this particular manner of making sounds, of making consonants.

Let us try to make a D. Now attempt to make the same movement with the legs: you hop, and while hopping you bend the legs somewhat at the knee. Here one must try to get the patients to bend at the knee and hop more and more powerfully and have them jump. Perhaps Mrs. Baumann will demonstrate the T for us; here the corresponding movement will be a hop forwards with an attempt at making knock-knees.* Thus while stepping forward you make the attempt to hop forwards and form knock-knees. That is what must be carried out. Our first concern is to demonstrate these things. So we have D and T. When one carries out the so-called soft sound one can remedy milder conditions, and with the so-called hard sound, the more severe conditions of this sort. Of course one must have the patients repeat them for several minutes until they are quite tired — in these things it is really a matter of carrying the exercise out until one is tired. And when one carries them out to fatigue, the

* X-beine; literally, X-legs.

D- and the T-sounds in particular are a force which works to strengthen the intestinal activity, particularly that activity which comes to expression in constipation. In this manner one can counteract constipation in many cases. Such a matter is unquestionably evident to the person who knows the physiological connections between the speech organism — which takes up the movement in the course of learning to speak — and the metabolic-limb system.

Now perhaps you will be so good, Miss Wolfram, and demonstrate the G-sound for us. Here is a matter of trying again to move forward in a similar manner while forming knock-knees. It would be the same thing with the K sound (Mrs. Baumann). And now you must try to hop forwards with the legs spread out sharply, with the Q as well; but that is the same thing again. Here in the case of G, as well as of K and of Q we have a movement which stimulates the forward motion, the inner mechanization of the intestine, which thus promotes the movement of the intestine itself. The difference in the physiological effect of D and T, G, K, and Q, is that in the case of D and T the processing of the food itself is more affected while with G, K, and Q the effect is more on the forward motion of the food in the intestine when the intestine itself lags.

Particularly important and therapeutically fruitful is the S. When you do the S-sound it is necessary to hop, to hop forwards keeping the legs continuously in the O-form, and to make the S-sound. Because one continually sets the legs down in this O-shape, namely, this actually has a very inward connection with the human digestive activity, and that is with the metabolic activity as it works back upon the entire human organism. In this movement one has something which one can have those children do who show an insufficent digestive activity and, who therefore, have headaches, since this movement regulates in particular the formation of gas in the intestine. When this is not in order, when it is either insufficient or too strong, this movement in particular will have a most important effect.

Then we have the F-sound. (Mrs. Baumann). One has to do here with something psychic. One must try to perform the jump in the following manner: one begins and tries to go forward; in landing one must come down hard on the tips of the toes, however, and now bring the heels down — once again, a jump onto the tips of the toes, then down on to the heels again. In the case of the V,* it would be just the same. Here we have a movement which should be practised when one finds that urination is not in order. It has a stimulative effect on the passing of urine. When it is necessary to animate this — for whatever reason — here is the movement to be performed.

It is, of course, entirely possible to combine the movements in the most varied manners; one will find in giving treatment that one will have to combine the one with the other — depending on the direction to be taken.

If we make an R (Miss Wolfram) I must ask you to please make it in such a way that in stepping forwards you always stretch distinctly, then with the left foot thus (here Dr. Steiner demonstrated the bending and stretching movement himself; the ed.), put the weight on the foot, stretch and as you step forwards — continuing in this manner to put the weight on the foot with the legs bent — you must try to make the R. That would have to be developed in this manner. If one were to practise this R with a person for a few minutes — one would have to practise it frequently during the day, however — it would regulate the rhythm of evacuation were that not in order. That is something which works directly over onto the rhythm of evacuation and regulates it.

Apart from its being necessary to do these movements not in a dilettantic fashion, but in a manner suitable to the matter at hand, in accordance with the diagnosis, it will be important for the observation of the whole dynamics of the

* V is pronounced in the same way as F in German.

human being to keep the connections which come thus to light in view.

Now an L, (Mrs. Baumann) here again together with the effort to place the legs in the knock-kneed position and hop forwards — draw together — now once again. It should be an effort to hop forwards, too. The forwards motion is entirely necessary in such a case. This movement works especially strongly on the peristalsis, on the movement of the intestine itself. With this movement one can also have the patient move backwards in the same manner. He will have much more difficulty in learning to do it, but it will have a significant effect in regulating the movement of the intestine itself, the peristalsis, as all these movements in fact work in a regulative manner out of the limb-metabolic system into what is in this connection a dependency of the limb-metabolic system (or at least adjacent to it) that is, into the circulation and into the respiratory movement as well.

A very interesting letter is the H, which actually has the most vowel nature attached to it. One should accompany the H in walking as follows: one tries to stand with the legs together, to hop forwards, and in the course of this hop forwards, to spread the legs and strike the floor with the legs apart; one should always be moving forwards. That is a movement which, I beg you to take notice, must be carried out thoroughly slowly, however. In the case of the other movements it is important to carry them out quickly; this movement, however, must be carried out slowly and there must be pauses for rest between each of the jumps as well. This must be taken into account with this movement as it has a very strong effect on the regulation of intestinal activity in the area of transition from the stomach into the intestine. Therefore, when one notices that someone cannot get his food from the stomach into the intestine, it will be greatly to his advantage to perform this movement, but, as I said, tranquilly and standing still after each separate hop.

Now we have the M. (Mrs. Baumann) This M must be

46

made with the "peewit step". It is good to do one step with one leg and the next with the other leg — forth and back. One can also do the peewit step backwards and then with the other leg forwards again. This technique of doing the peewit step backwards is something which one should really master. It is in fact a movement which it is important to study, then when the M is carried out in this form in movement it acts to regulate the entire metabolic system and limb system and it is extraordinarily important to practise it with the children during puberty. When this exercise with M is practised at the time of sexual maturity it will prove a strong regulator of over assertive sexuality. It will regulate over assertive sexuality when practised during puberty. One must only have developed an eye for whether it should be practised in this manner. It is not without reason the M was regarded as an especially important sound in the time when people still understood something of the inner content of the sounds; it is the sound which closes the OM syllable of the Orient. The OM syllable of the Orient is closed by M because the whole human being is in fact regulated through the metabolic-limb system by exactly this sound. Thus this movement is particularly regulatory. In the ancient culture it was customary to have the younger people perform such movements in order to educate them to be corporally complete human beings and, at the same time, reserved persons.

Then we have the N sound. The N-sound is accompanied by a jump in which the knees are bent from the beginning. So, one keeps the legs, the knees, bent and then jumps. That is a movement which strengthens the intestinal activity greatly and in such a manner that it can be applied where there is a tendency to diarrhoea. That can serve as a substantiation or as an indication of how one can see the effect of the system of movement on the metabolic system. That is something which one really only notices when one considers the connections between the system of movement and the metabolic system in the light of one's knowledge of the threefold order of the human organism. This threefold order

47

of the human organism sheds light in fact on many things; in our present time where knowledge of the soul consists almost solely of words, one can think out at length all sorts of exercises in which one believes one has taken the soul element into account — or one can develop gymnastics in which one takes only the bodily physiology into consideration. One can talk at length around and about these matters; without knowledge of the threefold order of the human organism one will not attain to any clarity in them. It was interesting, in fact, to have a physiologist of the present day here who listened to one of the introductions which I usually give at eurythmy performances and then saw eurythmy as well. Now I normally say that in education one will have to replace the sort of gymnastics that proceeds solely from physiology with this soul-filled sort of gymnastics. Thereupon the physiologist, who is also known as a very great authority in nutritional matters, said that for him it wasn't enough to say that one shouldn't overrate gymnastics; for him gymnastics was no method of education at all, but a barbarism.

Now, you see, behind something like this is hidden a very important symptom of the times. It is, on the one hand, just as correct to say that the gymnastics of today is usually one-sidedly conceived — since it is taken out of the physiology and anatomy of the organism alone — as it is at least one-sided on the other hand to say that gymnastics is a barbarism. Why? Because when one develops gymnastics out of the physiology of the body alone it becomes a barbarism. It is our materialistic education and civilization that first made a barbarism out of gymnastics. In the manner in which gymnastics is practised today, it is a barbarism. And this conception of gymnastics is connected with some completely false notions, is it not? For example, people believe — although the experts don't believe it anymore, still many people believe that if one has a person exert himself mentally* and then allows him to recover, as

* geistig

48

they believe, corporally thereafter, that constitutes a proper recuperation. But that isn't true at all! If a person does arithmetic or gymnastics for an hour he will become equally tired in reality; it makes no difference. That is known today, but people cannot properly judge how soul and spirit should be brought into gymnastic movements, how the movements carried out are to proceed from the human being as a whole. Now one will have to develop gymnastics gradually in such a way that what we are developing as artistic eurythmy can unite with what is thus developed as physiological gymnastics. And one can make the transition from the eurythmic to the gymnastic quite well. It will only be necessary to see that this sort of eurythmy which actually takes the part of a sort of soul-filled gymnastics in the course of instruction is done with humour; before everything else it must give the children delight. It must give the children joy; that is a part of it. To teach eurythmy like a grumpy, dried-out school-master would be something which could really not be done at all.

Now we still have the Sh. (Miss Wolfram) When it is accompanied by a small jump, then a larger jump, a small jump, then again a larger jump, a smaller jump, a larger jump, then one has a movement with a strong effect in the Sh as well; however, it too must be carried out slowly. It is not necessary to slow the N-movement down particularly, but with the H and Sh movement it is essential to do them slowly and in the case of the latter to take a short rest after every three jumps, at the transition to the next set; thus a rhythm is brought into it as well: short, long, short — and now one rests — long, short, long — and now a rest — short, long, short, — now a rest. Thus one has in this a movement which in the appropriate cases — one can combine movements, of course — affects the beginning portions of the intestinal tract, which pertains to the stomach. When someone has what is in itself such a weak digestion that the food remains

49

lying in the stomach — I have drawn attention to similar matters on other occasions — that will also be particularly the case where the H-movement is involved. with the Sh movement, however, one must notice, for example, whether stomach acid is easily produced and so on; then the Sh-movement should be carried out.

So you see the consonants as they are performed eurythmically are connected with the formation of man in a totally different manner from the eurythmic vowels. As we considered the making of vowels in eurythmy I had to draw your attention to the manner in which the inward, that which lies more to the interior, is related to movement. Here we have to do with the effect on the third member of the threefold organism.

Now when applying that which we discussed the day before yesterday in regard to the vowels, it would be good to have the patient sound the vowel of the exercise to be done, slowly, before the exercise as such is begun. So that without singing — singing would be of less help in this case — he very simply entones the sound at length, and when he has done this for a time, when he has sounded it out loud, one would have him carry out the movement for the vowel in question. When he has done that one should try to call forth in him the impression that he hears the sound that he has just carried out. You will find that in the present day only very few people have the impression that they hear the sounds inwardly in a soul-spiritual manner. Thus one must tell him to enter into a state of soul such as if he were to hear the "I". It is particularly important to understand this matter. Then, you see, when you have the patient speak the vowel, entone it, the organism as such feels as if the sound were being induced. If he then carries out the movement it appears to be the result of the spoken sound. And then one listens. One entones the "I", then does the movement, and then in one's fantasy imagines that one hears the "I" sounding. Then we have: the calling forth of the "I", that which arises through the movement of the "I", the hearing of that which has moved, the hearing of the sound once again. This is something which brings a great deal of life into this human etheric body; and in precisely those directions we have pointed out it brings real life into the etheric body. In these matters, in these exercises the intention is to bring movement into the human etheric body, to bring an inwardly regulated movement into the etheric activity of the human organism. It is particularly interesting to see how the movement, which as a movement of the intestine progresses from the front to the back, releases a movement in the etheric body which proceeds from back to front and then breaks on the abdominal wall — it does not actually break, but disappears. This latter movement is in most cases where the intestinal activity is not in order, in gross disorder as well. This activity which counters the physical movement will be aroused particularly by the R-movement, for example. Here there is a very lively vibrating from back to front and that is the element in the R-movement which affects the rhythm of elimination in a very specific manner.

It can also be used pedagogically as the whole human organism is a unity and everything in it works in a unitary fashion. If you were to survey children in school, for example, you would find amongst them some who can hardly pronounce an R, who are quite shocking in their pronunciation of the R. Of course, the factors can be crossed and the matter may not be self-evident — nevertheless, such children are always simultaneously candidates for constipation: one does them a kindness, in fact, by doing something such as I showed you yesterday with them: the R-movement, which affects the rhythm of evacuation positively. It is indeed possible to make use of these things pedagogically. One must only always have the indications and one must not go too far. The physician, however, can go much further as he will find that specific symptoms naturally appear when the exercise is practised for days and weeks. But he is, of course, in the position to counter these symptoms, which quite justifiably appear, by other means. I want to point out that if the effect of the N-movement were to become too predominant, one would only have to counteract it with the D-movement and one would nevertheless have achieved that which was to be achieved. Thus one can balance one by means of the other.

The only other thing I wish to say today is that I really do not want artistic eurythmy to be influenced in any way whatsoever by the discussion which must of course arise when eurythmy is considered as a hygienic-therapeutic discipline. I beg the artistic eurythmists to forget these things thoroughly when they practise artistic eurythmy so that they are not confused by their thoughts on digestive activity when they are involved in artistic eurythmy. That would be most troubling. One must nevertheless be entirely clear, however, that human art does have to do with the whole human being and does not proceed from the head alone. And especially in the case of an art of movement that must naturally be kept in view.

That is what I had as yet to tell you. In the following days we will discuss more what has to do with the evolution of man, with reference to what comes to the fore after certain intervals of time, that is to say, what occurs at a later age, as the consequence of an exercise affecting the organism of the child.

LECTURE 5

Dornach April 16, 1921

Today we will go over to some of those eurythmic exercises more related to the activity proceeding from the soul. Before we begin, however, it will be necessary to take note that it is usually assumed when a person produces an expression of will or when he arrives at a judgment, that these expressions are connected with the human nervous system alone. This, however, is not at all the case; one must make it clear to oneself that the judgments which the human being passes, for example, are bound up with his entire constitution; that man pronounces a judgment out of the totality of his being. Thus when one makes the eurythmic movement corresponding to a judgment, here again, the whole human being is influenced in a certain manner; it is not only the head which will be subject to the influences of what arises through judging eurythmically. Mrs. Baumann will show us the movement which corresponds to confirmation, and then the one corresponding to negation. Naturally it should be carried out several times without interruption when used as therapeutic exercise. Now this confirmation and negation is precisely that which can be called a judgment; when one confirms or negates something one has to do with the nature of judgment in its essence. When you give such a confirmation or negation, the movement works, when it is repeated frequently, by way of a detour through the etheric body very strongly on the respiratory system. One can by this means counter a tendency to shortness of breath. You can for example repeat the confirmation ten times consecutively, then the negation, and follow this up with confirmation, negation, confirmation,

53

negation — both ten times consecutively. Whatsoever illness this shortness of breath may be the symptom of, by this means one will be able to counteract it in such a way that the entire constitution is affected as the whole matter occurs by way of a detour through the etheric body. You must only keep in sight what is being done here. One could interpret what Mrs. Baumann has done touching upon what is essential in it as follows: what she projects thereby into the world is a thought that has become fleeting, a thought which has gained wings and gone over into movement. When a judgment is fixed eurythmically — as a confirmation or negation — then it is a thought which rides on the movement. And because the thought rides on the movement one projects in fact on the one hand, a part of this being outwards; on the other hand, because the thought rides on the movement one takes a part more thoroughly into oneself than otherwise. That is to say, one makes a movement through which one becomes more awake than one otherwise is. Such movements are actually movements that awaken. However, because one does not wake up with the ego at the same time in the same manner, the activity of the ego is in a certain way dampened. This dampening of the ego is not absolute, however, but in relation to the organism. In fighting shortness of breath by means of this detour through the etheric body this constitutes what would be the first symptom reached and what is introduced into the whole human constitution by means of the by-way through the etheric body.

Now a disposition of the will*: sympathy and antipathy. Now imagine you make this movement repeatedly, one after another: sympathy, antipathy, sympathy, antipathy, or only one of these two. When one does this, in a certain sense one is setting out something which one carries within oneself; naturally this can only be confirmed through observation. It is a sort of falling asleep. The other movement (confirmation and negation; the ed.) must be carried out quickly, and this

* Willenszustimmung

54

must be carried out slowly. It is indeed a movement which brings forth the imagination of sleep in the observer; imaginatively one falls asleep in a way with such a movement — not in reality, however, at least that shouldn't happen. But because one in reality doesn't go to sleep while making this movement, the "I" is more strongly active in relation to the body than it usually is. And by means of such a movement the circulation and the digestion as a whole are stimulated. The entire digestion is really stimulated in such a manner that through such a movement the tendency to belch, for example, can be counteracted.

Now we want to express that which one could call the feeling of love towards something (Mrs. Baumann). Take a good look at this, the feeling of love for something. Imagine it carried out ten times consecutively and accompanied by a powerful E between each of the movements. Thus, Love-E, Love-E, and so on, one after another. You accompany the movements which you have learned as expressing feeling in eurythmy — it could be another feeling as well — with the movement for E. Here we have a strong influence which proceeds from the human etheric to act on the astral nature and which has the effect of warming the circulation. It is something which really works on the circulatory system in a beneficial manner. One cannot say that it accelerates or retards the circulation; it affects it in a beneficially warming manner.

We also have something which could be called a wish: Hope. (Miss Wolfram) Look at this and picture to yourself that one carries out this movement for the wish repeatedly — always returning to the position of balance, then carrying out the movement for the wish again — and always alternating it with the movement for U. This means that the astral will act very strongly upon the etheric and it can be said that a beneficial warming effect on the breathing system will result. Naturally one must take into consideration that all these things of which we have spoken today occur by way of the etheric body and can, therefore, never show what effect they have on the following day. Some effects may appear after two to three days and are then, however, all the more certain.

Now imagine that we make a bending and stretching movement with the legs and at the same time a definite B-movement (Mrs. Baumann). That which I have just shown you simultaneous with a decided B movement, now rest, B while bending, ten times consecutively. That is something which people who very frequently have migraine or other headaches should do. The time for them to do it, however, is not when they have the headache, but rather when they do not.

A particularly effective movement is the following: bend and stretch the torso forwards and backwards accompanying this movement simultaneously with the movement for R. (Miss Wolfram) Bend forwards, bend backwards with the R; that consecutively and often. That affects the whole rhythmic system, the rhythm of breathing and of circulation, positively. When there are irregularities present there, this will work extraordinarily well under all conditions.

Now I will ask you to take a look at another most effective movement which consists in shaking the head to the right and left with the movement for M. The head should not be turned, in so far as possible, but only bent to the right and left, and that with the M-movement. That is something which when practised has a very strong quieting effect on all possible irregularities in the lower body, again by way of the etheric body. Irregularities in the lower system which express themselves through pains can be mitigated thereby. One must combat tendencies to such pains when the pains are not present. That is the crux of the matter. While the pains are present it cannot very well be carried out. The important thing is to carry it out so long as the pains are not present.

Please take note of the following: strike the knee with the foot, stemming the movement of the foot against the knee;

picture this accompanied by an E movement with the arms. It is a very beautiful movement. It can and should be carried out as an exercise with children in school, as when it is done frequently it wages war against the most varied aspects of clumsiness. The children will at least be well cured of their clumsiness when they practise just this exercise. And when the children come and say that their shoulders hurt so and everything possible hurts, then you should reply: that is exactly what I wanted; you will be especially glad about it once it's better again! Every pain that is brought about in this manner combats clumsiness. Thus in respect to this one can deal quite energetically with the children.

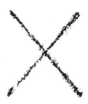

Now we will take a look at another variety (of movement). Imagine every sort of E movement which can be carried out with the arms now projected onto the floor. This movement comes into existence when this line crosses the other at an angle. Now let us imagine it in this way: Mrs. Baumann places herself here, Miss Wolfram there. Now walk and accompany the whole thing with an E movement with the arms. Run so that you pass by one another, but pay attention that you don't run into each other. So you make an E on the floor and an E with the arms and you pay attention at the same time that you don't collide. It is this taking notice of the other person, this exerting of one's concentration on him combined with the E-gesture which works together with the movement here. This exercise can only be carried out with two people. It is — when carried out by two people — essentially what one would call a strengthening of the heart, all that which is connected with the phenomena which one generally terms the strengthening of the heart.

Question: Could one have this exercise carried out by one sick and one healthy person?

One can readily do that, but one would perhaps have to have the healthy person omit the E-movement with the arms. This movement is especially intended for the clinical situation where one will, of course, have two people in need of a strengthening of the heart; it really is better if one has two such people.

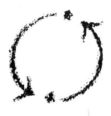

Now let us imagine the movement so: one of the ladies stands here, the other here, behind one another. When you arrive here, then Miss Wolfram carries out the path which you have begun, but in such a manner that she is always facing forwards. Then as the movement carries on, you take this part of the path and you the other. You initiate the continuation of your own movement in the other person and accompany it with the O position of the arms. Now one must see that the people who do this begin at a certain tempo; to begin with it must be slower, then become ever faster and faster. This rapid tempo should then ebb out into a slower one. That is then a movement which serves to strengthen the diaphragm significantly and thereby the whole breathing system. Here again, when one leaves out the O movement with the arms one can have a healthy person participate, but it is of course best to employ two people who are in need of healing.

Now I will ask you, Mrs. Baumann, to demonstrate the H movement for us once again. And now I will ask you to make this movement in such a way that you hold the arms still and imitate the movement with the shoulders alone as well as possible. In this case, however, one must accustom oneself to doing this movement with the shoulders and making an A with the arms at the same time, an A of any sort with the arms. That should be repeated frequently. You see, that is what could be designated as: "laughing eurythmically". That is how one laughs eurythmically. And when one laughs thus eurythmically that which one has in the curative effect of laughing itself is really very greatly heightened. The curative effect of laughing is well known. But when one practises laughing eurythmically, this curative effect is proportionately greater. You could do it otherwise as well, however.

Miss Wolfram, please make an A movement of some sort. And now try to make the same movement I spoke of before, the shoulder movement of the H, but do it quite slowly as if you wished to do it thoughtfully. Thus into the A movement of the arms one makes the shoulder movement of the H. One could designate that as follows: the whole organism is brought into accord with the feeling of veneration. It encompasses all that which the feeling of veneration actually effects in the organism. The effect on the human organism of the feeling of veneration, when it is habitual, is to make the organism as such actually more durable, more sturdy. It becomes capable of greater resistance. People who really have the capacity for veneration inherent in them become more capable of resistance within their organism. That is why everything which brings children to veneration, to the gift or capacity for reverence makes children more resistant. And one can come to the assistance of this capacity for resistance through this last eurythmic exercise.

One must keep in mind that what we have demonstrated today as decision, expression of will, hope, love, what we have shown in respect to certain organic pains, what we have demonstrated as a means of combating clumsiness and so on, all these things are related to man in such a way that the human being is gripped through them in the innermost part of his organic being and by way of a detour through the etheric body actually derives the possibility of making this etheric body into a workable instrument. The etheric body is a part of man which becomes stiff in most of those people who sit out their lives, spend their lives without interest for their surroundings. And it is not good when the human etheric body becomes stiff; nor for the organic functions is it good. When one has the exercises which we have described today carried out by children in moderation and by the appropriate patients very energetically (one can see by the indications given which patients have need of them), the etheric body will become supple and inwardly flexible. And by means of them one will do the children as well as the adults a good service.

These movements are indeed such that one can give them priority over the usual gymnastic movements; the usual gymnastic movements are taken in reality from the physiology, from the physis of the body alone and they tear the physical body continually out of the etheric body. Thus, the physical body then makes its own movements which do not pull the movements of the etheric body in the appropriate manner after them. For this reason the usual, merely physiologic, gymnastics is basically a school for materialism, since by means of it materialistic thought is transformed into feeling. Eurythmy makes man capable of recognising himself within increasingly and of gaining control over himself inwardly. Therefore such exercises have a pedagogic-didactic value as well as therapeutic and hygienic value. The attempt should be made to have these exercises — those described today, I mean — carried out by adults as well in moderation and to develop them in such a way that they could be carried out by the sick in a clinical situation.

A question has been put to me which could perhaps lead to something — and some other questions as well. Here is the question: "The Chinese cannot pronounce the letter R, they substitute L for it. Strawberries thus becomes stlawbellies, for example. Does that have to do with their race?"

It has to do with the organisation of the organism insofar as that is racially determined, of course. Through the particular gift of one part of mankind for one sound or another one can see what tendencies are inherent in certain people by virtue of their race. I brought such things to discussion just a few hours ago.

Other questions have been put about exercises which could be used in relation to conditions of indolence, insufficient reaction, lethargy and so on; conditions which frequently have to do with an insufficient thyroid activity. And here it has been brought to our attention that Fliess, in his well-known book about the course of life, has placed this complex of symptoms in the intermediate sexual category. How could a contemporary author not do so? Everything about which he knows very little he chalks up to the intermediate sexual category, or some other way. He puts the left-handed, for example, in the same category. I want to emphasize, expressly, however, that I have never recommended a eurythmic exercise with a special right-left emphasis to anyone.

(Attention was drawn to the exercises which one should begin either to the right or to the left: iambus, trochee.)

That is not in order to particularly accentuate an emphasis on the right or left, but rather in order to call forth the feeling of the iambus or trochee within the forward motion. That is thoroughly justified. The fact is that it has less to do with the long-short than it has to do with the particular movement. It is quite correct; it has to do with the fact that what lives in the breathing system is reversed when it is transferred into the system of movement. The upper man and the lower man are the reverse of one another. Thus every imaginable iambus in the breathing system, brought forth in speech, must of necessity become a trochee in the movement of legs and vice versa. Eurythmy in its entirety is based on this principle. You may test the whole of eurythmy in respect to it: eurythmy does not follow the principle of similarity in its execution, but the movement which is in keeping with the polar image. It is all entirely in accord with the image formed as the other polarity. This idea must be maintained throughout. But I have never recommended to anyone that he do something especially right or left; that should be left completely to the feeling. The question of whether a thing should be done with the right hand or the left hand should be determined only by those matters which would otherwise come into consideration. I do not want people to have the impression that I would have suggested an emphasis on the right in particular eurythmic exercises to any more left-sided person whosoever. That is not the case.

In addition I would like to emphasize the following. It is the case that when one has to do with insufficient reaction or with lethargy this more general indication will fall into some category which I have already given; lethargy is a general expression and can be relegated to something or other about which I have spoken. The appropriate movements should then be carried out.

On the whole one should see that with an exercise such as I have just given in connection with judgment and expression of will* — that the appearance of indolence, of lethargy and so on can be combatted very especially by that which I have given for the expression of will. And if one should notice that this is not particularly effective, one can alternate that exercise with the exercise that I have given for judgment, but in such a way that one attempts to discover — as it is here a

* Willensäusserung

question of trial — whether it is more effective when one varies the expression of will and the expression of judgment in a ratio of three to two or of two to three — one shorter, the other longer. And since these things work by way of a detour through the etheric body, one will find that one will first have to begin and carry on with these exercises for two to three days and according to the circumstances — when one sees that they are not having the proper effect — make a change on the third day. But in general one can say that the one exercise so well as the other will have an awakening effect on man in both directions. The will exercise and the judgment exercise are thus the ones that come into particular consideration.

In order that there be no misunderstanding, I emphasize that of course the opinion must not arise that these exercises would have a very significant effect after being carried out for two or three days. That would be an error. In order to produce an effect, these exercises should be carried out for at least seven weeks. Thus one can maintain — without necessarily being mystically inclined — that the space of time necessary for the beneficial effects just described to show themselves would be about seven weeks.

That is what I wanted to tell you today concerning these matters. I would like to request that the corresponding session tomorrow follow the other directly, after a short pause. Tomorrow will be the last eurythmy session then, as it will be necessary to have two purely medical sessions one after the other on Monday.

LECTURE 6

Dornach, April 17, 1921

There is so unendlessly much one could relate about the connection between the hygienic-therapeutic and eurythmy. Today we want to take into consideration that part of the physiological which we discover in the proximity of the spiritual when we contemplate a eurythmic exercise. Of course, all that which can be observed in this connection in artistic eurythmy will be encountered in an intensified form when one makes the transition from artistic eurythmy to the fortified eurythmy we have become acquainted with in these days. Nevertheless, the essence of that which concerns us can already be discovered purely artistically in a performance of eurythmy and the physiology corresponding to it then sought out. Let us try this by carrying out the following.

Perhaps Mrs. Baumann will be so good and perform the poem "Über allen Gipfeln ist Ruh" alternately in vowels and in consonants, while you (Frau Dr. Steiner) recite it.

Now let us make clear to ourselves what is taking place here, proceeding however very exactly. What is happening? A poem is recited. The person who does the eurythmy listens — he is the one who comes for us into consideration physiologically. That is the first matter of importance. He doesn't speak himself, he listens. That is essential. He listens to something which is in essence the meaningful word, a meaningful association of words. He listens to something in which the activity of thought and of mental representation are alive. What he perceives outwardly is the activity of mental representation clothed in an association of sounds. That is something which man in his waking, day-time existence often

64

does, is it not? But what actually takes place when he does it? If you consider the process from a psychologic-physiologic point of view you will easily discover that a light, partial sleep overtakes the listener. The "I" and the astral body glide over what they are taking in, they live into it. In listening man steps out of himself slightly. He is overcome by a condition which is similar and then again dissimilar to sleep. It is similar to sleep in that the "I" and astral body are slightly disengaged, dissimilar in that they remain receptive, perceptive and self-aware. Thus the process is extraordinarily similar to imagination. It is a subtle, conscious imagining that is still strongly suppressed in the subconscious. Such is the process at hand.

To every such process is a reaction within the human being himself; we take this into account as well. Let us look at what takes place in the person who is not reciting. What does he do when he listens? He brings his etheric body into motion. The etheric body reacts. In fact the etheric body takes up those movements which it carries out — only much more weakly — when the person is asleep and has left his etheric body behind in the physical body. When the human being is asleep the etheric body is considerably more active than when he is awake. During this dampened sleep taking place in the listener the movements of the etheric body are awakened to a greater degree. These movements of the etheric body can be observed. Thus in the listener one has a person demonstrating in a heightened manner the movements which the human being carries out otherwise in a a weakened form in sleep. Thus you can study in the listener, who promptly performs them for you, ether movements of the human being in sleep. It isn't at all necessary to study the person while asleep; one can study the etheric movements of the human being when listening and has in fact here the heightened movements of the etheric body in sleep. One studies these movements and has them carried out by the physical body. That is to say one allows the physical body to glide into all those etheric movements which one has studied in the manner just described. Thus in eurythmy one does what the human being carries out with his etheric body constantly while listening. You can see what is actually taking place.

Now that we have observed what actually occurs, its effect will become apparent as well. The result is that by means of the physical movement one carries over into consciousness what otherwise occurs unconsciously. One stimulates the astral body and the ego by means of this detour through the physical body and strengthens them. But what happens as a result of this? When the astral body and the ego are strengthened in this manner their activity becomes similar to the activity in the child and still growing person as it occurs naturally. You are calling upon the forces of growth in the human being. You are working directly into the person's forces of growth. If the person is still a child and shows signs of being retarded in his growth, you can stimulate his growth in this way. If the person is no longer a child, and the forces of growth have already diminished, or if the person is actually in the second half of his life, one calls upon the youthful forces, the rejuvenating forces in him which, however, cannot contribute to his growth since the human organism is, of course, fully developed. We can expedite a child in his growth or combat his abnormal growth by having him do eurythmy. In the case of the fully-grown person the inner organism presents too great a resistance to the outer organism for us to be able to make him grow. Nevertheless, we can still introduce these forces of growth. The result is that they crash against the resistance of organism and metamorphose; that means that they activate in their metamorphosed state the plastic force of the inner organs. They stimulate the plastic force of the inner organs and these inner organs learn to breathe better and to better digest. They are encouraged to fulfil the necessary activity of the human organism in its entirety.

66

When artistic eurythmy is performed one should not think of it in the first instance as curative eurythmy; nevertheless, in the moment a person begins to be abnormal in any way it will have a curative effect. We have already seen the examples where when the usual eurythmy is reinforced, the reaction which follows is naturally also strengthened and we can form a mental picture of how this eurythmy affects the plastic qualities of the organization.

You can understand that the habitual practise of eurythmy activates the plasticity of the organs, thier plastic force, and that as a result the human being becomes internally a better breather, a better person, if I may express myself so, in respect to his inwardly oriented digestion. He becomes a person who has his whole organism more within his own discretion. He becomes an inwardly more agile person. And to become a true artist is nothing other than to make the inner man more flexible, plastic, agile. That can be seen when one sculpts, for example. One cannot sculpt properly if in experience one cannot transpose oneself for example into the figure that one is developing plastically, if one cannot bring to life in oneself the forces that are building the figure, that express themselves in the figure. If, however, one sees the human organism itself as an implement and carries out what corresponds within, then what is the case in outward artistry is in a higher degree the case here as well for at this point one can do nothing other than to call forth internally what corresponds to the outward movement.

If you would be so good we will do the poem again now, this time with only the vowels. So that the emphasis is on the vowels alone. (Miss Wolfram and Frau. Dr. Steiner)

What I have just said about the physiology of eurythmy is specialized here. When only the vowels are carried out then that which I have characterized does not come to expression in its entirety. What I characterized is correct when someone speaks and the movements for consonants and vowels are made alternately. For what we have just done is that which I said not entirely correct: it will have to be specialized. Here very specific, differentiated movements have been performed all of which prove to be movements within the etheric body having primarily to do with what lies in the rhythmic system. Thus we must fasten our attention on that system which — as an etheric system — participates especially when vowels are spoken. When a person listens to vowels — which occurs of course in so specialized a manner only in eurythmy and to which for this reason attention must be drawn as it is here especially important therapeutically — when one recites a simple sequence of vowels for this person, or when one has him carry out such movements, in which case he would be listening to the movements which are the forms of expression for the vowel element while doing eurythmy — then, in the normal person listening to vowels those movements of the the etheric body corresponding to the rhythmic system become active in the way described earlier. And now you have the person doing eurythmy carry out in turn those movements through which he glides with his physical body into the movements which are otherwise manifest in the etheric body when vowels are heard. That is how the matter is specialized. In this way in particular those organs which belong to the rhythmic system are stimulated to respiration and inward digestion. These organs are strengthened; in them the appeal goes out to the forces of growth in the growing child or to the plastic forces which have their resistance within the organization of the fully grown adult.

This will serve as an introduction to the physiology of the vowels in eurythmy. Thus in applying to therapeutic ends everything derived from the vowel-element in eurythmy you will be able to affect the rhythmic organs in particular.

Now perhaps Mrs. Baumann will do the same poem once again consonantally. A mere glance will testify to the radical difference between the consonants and the vowels as they are carried out eurythmically. The difference is indeed thoroughly radical. If we wish to study what we have just seen we will have to make clear to ourselves how the matter would lie if in ordinary listening we were to hear only the consonants. For civilized man that is seldom so, but among less civilized peoples it is sometimes the case that they must listen to much of a consonantal nature. The consonantal world in speech is appreciably richer among less civilized peoples, and the transition from one consonant to another is stronger and unilluminated by a vowel lying between. You will find it possible to observe this up to and even within Europe. Just look at words written in the Czech language and you will see just what combinations of consonants are present. To be sure when the words are spoken the vowel element sounds within these combinations of consonants, but it permeates them only as a continuous, hardly differentiated undercurrent. And if you listen to Czech you will say to yourself: to listen to this consonantal element is entirely different from listening to a language that is thoroughly permeated by vowels. Thus one has to do with quite another process here which can be characterized best in the following manner.

As an ordinary listening process this process calls forth strongly those movements of the etheric body which are otherwise actually carried out in the case of physical movements. They are retained and so, while listening to consonants, the human being lives in a certain tension. Unconsciously he would like to be imitating outwardly, physically, when he listens to consonants, but he holds back. The situation is alive with tension: a state of pacification prevails, but an artificially induced pacification, called forth by the power of one's own ego in opposition to those movements which demand to be carried out. Volition dammed up within itself is manifest when consonants are heard. Therefore you will find that listening to consonants is inwardly exceptionally invigorating. If one has an eye for it one can study how peoples such as the Czechs comport themselves inwardly — how the human being deports himself in his interior in relation to these tensions, these aggressive forces once one knows that they are built up out of the consonantal element of the language. It is a continual curbing of what unceasingly strives to become physical movement.

Once again it is for the human being a stepping-out, a going over into the condition of sleep, and this going out, this transition into sleep is extraordinarily interesting. Consider the human being schematically: head, rhythmic system, limb-metabolic system. In listening to consonants it is primarily the limb-metabolic system that is engaged. The person wants to move his limbs, wants to break into movement, but the movement is converted into tension. He passes as it were into a state of sleep which actually does not take place in other respects, for the ego and the astral body — which go out in ordinary sleep — remain within the organism. One even tries to bring about a sort of artificial sleep for the limb-metabolic system in this case. But when one falls asleep in the limb-metabolic system to a degree, a strong reaction makes itself evident. This reaction consists of dreaming. However, at the moment one's consciousness is not so organized that one can dream. Dreams come into being that play about the human being. (orange). They affect the outer astrality and the outer ether. People who listen to consonants reinforce the aura in their proximity. This expresses itself in turn in its polarity: what remains here in the subconscious as polar content plays about the head as a volition-feeling factor and penetrates into the organism of the head. (violet). Therefore you may notice an intensification of wilfulness and caprice in people who are accustomed to living in the consonantal element. Dreams transformed into will play through the organism of the head.

What are dreams transformed into will from a physiological point of view? If one examines the etheric-physical correlative, it is essentially what is plastically at work in the organization of the head. The plastic effect on the organization of the head is pre-eminent and in this manner it will be possible to

70

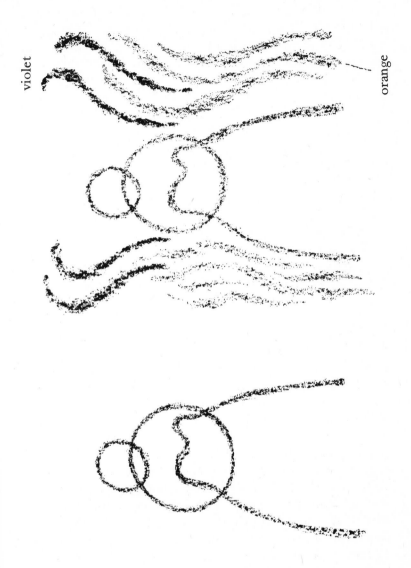

activate to a degree the organization of a head which is retarded. If one has to do with a feeble-minded person, or with someone where it can be demonstrated physically that his head organism is not in order, one should let him do consonants in eurythmy.

Then one engages oneself with those forces which otherwise work as dream-like will in the entire remaining limb-metabolic system, which stimulate there the organization and preserve its activity. One makes the heads of imbeciles and those who are otherwise retarded in their head-organization more active. Thus one can employ this sort of eurythmy to arouse curative forces for the organization of the head, particularly when one carries it out in the intensified form, with the strengthened form of the consonants of which we have heard in the last few days. It is natural that when one wishes to consider the physiology of eurythmy one should keep the active moving human being in view. In ordinary physiology one actually does not pursue physiology at all: even when an experiement is conducted on the living one proceeds from the mechanical; or one starts with the corpse and draws conclusions about physiology in actuality. One then arrives at something which one has inferred. If one wishes to attain to a physiology of these processes, what one otherwise infers must be read from inner activity of man. And it will be seen how this sort of study will quicken the whole of physiology. Consider alone the following: what is the process of digestion as observed in the living human being? It is metabolic activity which thrusts itself into the rhythmic activity, which unfolds in the direction of the rhythmic. Digestive activity is metabolic activity which is caught up to a degree by the rhythm of the circulatory organs. A continuing process, which is a combination of the metabolic activity and rhythmic activity (completed by the German editor) is taking place here. When the rhythm pulses up against it, what is metabolic activity in the lymph is caught up into the rhythm of the organs of circulation and pulled along with it. The more chaotic activity — the chaos astir in the movement of the lymph — is taken over into the rhythm of the circulatory system. Physically human volition lives there where the chaos of the lymph goes over into the regular rhythmic functioning of the circulatory system. One must distinguish this activity of will, which consists in the continual transition taking place between the chaotic vigour in the lymph and the rhythmically regular, harmonising activity present in the circulatory being, from the outer activity into which it however pours. It is, nevertheless, in this way that the inner world of man lying within the skin brings itself into harmony with the outer being of man. Through the subordination of his personal being man encorporates himself into the being of the outer world. Therefore, when one influences this activity through eurythmy — as we have seen with the consonants — one counters in fact the human being's tendency to become self-willed, to become egoistic, and his tendency to become organically egoistic as well. What does it actually mean when man becomes egoistic? Organically expressed it means that the force of plasticity in the organs is diminished and the rigidifying, crystallizing tendency takes the upper hand. The organs no longer want to be modellers, they want to become more crystalline. By means of consonantal eurythmy this tendency can be counteracted.

Here you have an insight deep into the human organism. Egoists are always people whose organs threaten to take on a proper wedge form. They want to become wedges, to become crystalline, where as in the case of people who are pathologically self-less, these organs expand. They have no crystallizing agency; they have plastic forces and become round. That is also a pathological condition. It is always the swing of the pendulum from one extreme to the other to which one must pay heed.

Consider what spiritual activity is: when man thinks and from out of his thinking feels — that is designated spiritual activity in normal life. It is carried out by the most physical part of the head organism and is for precisely this reason the sublimating spiritual activity, the individualizing on the one side, the abstractly felt on the other. When the human being carries out this activity, what happens then? He draws out of his organism the force that enables him to encorporate himself into the outer world. He draws out of himself the force that, pathologically, entices him to expand. He makes a crystallizer of himself when he is spiritually active. Certain peoples, the more northern peoples in particular, have developed a strong instinctive consciousness of these matters. Today they have as yet no inclination to introduce eurythmy in accordance with this instinctive consciousness. They employ instead what is more outwardly physiologic, Swedish gymnastics and so on. Nevertheless they make decided use of the characteristic alternating effect, by alternating the activity which the children must carry out in scientific study in school — when they must think and so on — with what diverts them to movement. They expect every teacher to be a gymnastic teacher as well and require on the other hand that the gymnastic instructor stands at the spiritual level of the child. Such things should be taken into consideration in an advanced civilization. However if I may make a statement that may appear to be a bit nasty, but is really meant only to enlighten, one must have time if one wishes to take these matters into account instinctively. Such things must be carried out by those peoples who take less part in the process of civilization, who live a life apart, more for themselves, and who are thus able to gradually develop instinctively that which has to do with the rhythm of spiritual and physical activity. The Swedes and the Norwegians who lead a more isolated existence, for example, can put such ideas into practice instinctively particularly well. For others the practice of such matters must be more conscious since these peoples are more engaged in the world processes in general — people, for example, who must concern themselves — as was of late very much the case — with making war and so on. These peoples must see these matters much more consciously. And those nations that stand in the centre of the world's movement, who must take part in its affairs while the world turns around them so to speak, they will soon see what they will get themselves into if they do not turn to these things consciously, how they will gradually degenerate. That is something which Switzerland in particular should take to heart.

These things can be observed to play a part in the state of the world as a whole. The general conditions prevailing in the world are, of course, the result of human activity and even today they proceed more from unconscious human activity than from conscious activity. We are given the task, however, to gradually transmute the unconscious activity of man into conscious activity.

How does this spiritual activity work in man? It awakens the crystallizing forces. In people with weak egos it strengthens the "I", it makes the ego more egoistic. In people who effuse organically because they are not sufficiently egoistic we will find it necessary to activate the forces of egoism — not for the benefit of the soul, but for the body. We could stimulate them by outward means as well; it would be natural to advise people who effuse organically to consume substances containing sugar. However, they sometimes have an antipathy towards them — a fact which gives expression to the true state of affairs.

However, that is something of much less interest to us at the moment. What interests us just now is that through the vowel element in eurythmy one has the possibility of working most effectively in this direction; one can bring the human being organically to himself through the vowels. One can awaken the forces which bring him to himself organically. For certain people that will be most necessary, among them the sleepyheaded people. One will find that the alternation between the two, between the vowels and the consonants in eurythmy, will work favourably as well as it enduces a living rhythm in the human being such as should exist between opening oneself to the world and retracting into oneself. That will be called forth by alternating consonantal and vowel elements in eurythmy.

It is, of course, particularly important, when one intends to apply eurythmy for therapeutic purposes, to make one's own what I would like to call this physiologic-psychologic perception of what actually takes place. One should understand that the person who does consonantal eurythmy tends to call forth around himself a sort of aura which works back on him and brings him out of an egoless mingling with the world; in the case of the person who does vowels in eurythmy, his aura is drawn together, densified in itself, which is, of course, always the case with spiritual activity as well, and that the inner organs are thus stimulated to bring the person to himself.

Pedagogically considered, alternating between the lessons one would place more in the morning hours where more mental work would be done and the lessons in which there would be more movement and where a great deal of eurythmy would be done calls forth rhythmic activity in the growing child that has an extraordinarily beneficial effect; all the detriments that are of necessity incurred through an improportionate mental exertion are balanced out again by doing eurythmy. For this reason eurythmy has an especially beneficial function within the curriculum as a whole.

That which I have to say about eurythmy particularly to the physicians I will convey in the course of my lectures to them. Thus we conclude our consideration of eurythmy as such here. Tomorrow there will be two consecutive medical lectures where the eurythmists are not present.

LECTURE 7

Dornach, April 18, 1921   (held before physicians)

In respect to particulars you will find it necessary to elucidate what I have to tell you today about eurythmy through your knowledge of physiology and so on. How that can be done will reveal itself to you as if of its own accord, if I may say so. When we look into a spiritual-corporeal process such as that which takes place in eurythmy, we may do no less than to indicate the deeper spiritual-physical connections as well. Thus I would like to draw your attention to the following.

First we must contemplate that extra-human world process which one usually traces only in its details and not in regard to what is actually inwardly active. Just consider what earth formation is, in reality: a formative tendency works from the planetary sphere inward. And furthermore, from what lies without the planetary sphere a formative working into the earth takes place: continuous, radiant cosmic forces revealing themselves in the individual potentialities ("Kraftentitäten", entities of force) radiating towards the earth.

In this connection we may conceive of these cosmic powers as working centripetally and building up that which is on and in the Earth from without — although they encompass all that I have said about such rays previously as well. The fact is that the metals of the Earth as a whole, for example, are not in essence formed out of some force or another within the Earth, but are actually set into the Earth from the Cosmos. Now these forces that work through the ether can be called formative forces, formative forces working in from outside and not from the planets, for in that case they would work towards the centre; the planets are there for the specific

77

purpose of modifying them, that is, the planetary sphere. Please take note of them in precisely this context: the formative forces. In opposition to them stand those forces in the human being and in the earth which take up those formative forces and make them fast, which assemble them around a point so that the earth can come into being. Those forces which make secure we may thus call the consolidating forces ("Kräfte des Befestigens") (please see the following diagram, and the one shown on page 81.)

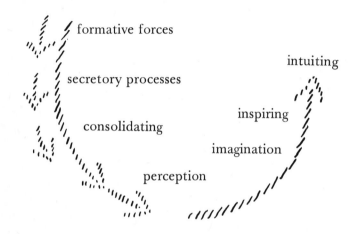

formative forces

secretory processes

consolidating

intuiting

inspiring

imagination

perception

In the human being they are present as the forces that build up the organs plastically, whereas the other forces, the formative forces, have more to do with propelling the organs out of the spiritual-etheric world into the physical world. That is a process which becomes so tangible in the contrast between the propulsive powers of magnesium and the rounding-off forces of fluorine. It is a process active every-where: in the teeth from below upwards and rounding-off at the top, but from front to back as well and from the back forwards, from above to below, rounding-off at the bottom. This process will become directly tangible if you picture to yourself that, in association with the tendency to push something spherical forwards, from without inwards, something is formed which is opposed by a process of spherical formation from below upwards (red, in the following illustration).

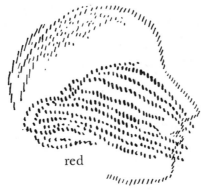

red

Between these two processes is that which mediates: processes of secretion and on the other hand, the absorption of what the other has secreted and so on, that which can be called processes of secretion in the widest sense; then in the final analysis absorption is dependent upon a secretion inwards which is in turn re-absorbed. In between lies thus what can be best called secretory processes.

Such a secretory process becomes tangible when you picture to yourself that on the one side lies what continually wants to secrete carbon (orange, in the illustration) and that which takes it up through respiration from the fore in the formation of carbon dioxide (white).

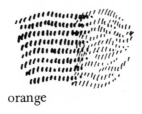

orange

Behind this such a process of secretion is taking place. When you descend further into the metabolic-limb system, you have a proper process of consolidation. However, this process is present in the other direction as well. You will be able to follow it most tangibly by studying the eye, which is built inwards from without, as embryology demonstrates, but is consolidated from within. The formation is internalized. That is the manner in which the eye develops. It is internalized (see the following drawing: orange).

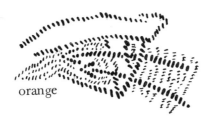

orange

Thus, as we progress to that which is of soul-spiritual nature in man, to the organs of the soul-spiritual, to the sense-organs, we find that the process of consolidation has become spiritualized, truly ensouled and spiritualized in perception; that is, more or less, the descending process which leads to the formation of the organs (please refer to the first illustration and to the chart which follows).

Thus we find at the lowermost end the process of sensory perception, objective perception. If this development continues, if it goes further in this direction, then the process of perception encounters the consolidating forces; should it become conscious in this encounter, it will become imagination. If imagination develops further and becomes conscious in encountering the process of secretion, it becomes inspiration. And when inspiration develops further in the direction of the formative forces, collides with them consciously and thus sees through these forces, it becomes intuition. Thus one can develop this progression in the life of the soul stage by stage from objective sensory perception to imagination, to inspiration and to intuition.

Formative forces
                        Intuition
Secretory processes
                        Inspiration
Consolidation
                        Imagination
            Perception

This process which unfolds in the soul is based, however, on the process of coming-into-being. It is in fact, as you can see here, only the inverse of this genesis. One steps out to encounter what has already come into existence, rising into this becoming in the opposite direction. Formation takes place in the descending direction. The human being ascends in the opposite direction; he advances to meet what is coming into being. Thus, what one develops as powers of perception and cognition in imagination, inspiration and intuition always has its counter-activity in the creative powers which express themselves in the formative forces, in the processes of secretion and consolidation.

From all of this you will gather that what is active in the human organism in the opposite direction, in its coming into being, is that into which one ascends when rising in knowledge. You will perceive that in reality what we attain in imagination are the same powers which, without our being conscious of them, reveal themselves in the phenomena of growth, in the plastic phenomena of growth. If we ascend to inspiration, we come upon the forces which inspire man from without inwards in his breathing, which shape him through and through as he breathes, which shape themselves into the plastic forces as they work these forces through, to a degree. And if we ascend to intuition, we rise in reality to the primal mover ("Agens") who enters into our plastic forms from the world without as substantial being.

81

You see, in this way we grasp the human being as he takes shape out of the Cosmos. If we now apply the knowledge which we have gained in one way or another through anatomy or physiology and illuminate it with what is given us here, then we begin to understand the organs and their functions. This is an indication of how to understand the organs and their functions. Thus what is always at work plastically in the human being, what permeates and shapes him, lives on the other hand in the movements for the consonants, the unconscious imaginative forces which call forth a permeation of the organism, as I said yesterday. Yesterday's lecture should be of help. Here you can perceive how consonantal eurythmy takes hold of deficient formative powers, deficient plastic forces in the human being and transforms them into something truly sculptural.*

Let us assume we have a child before us and we see that he is insufficiently formed,* that his growth* is rampant. What does it mean, when we say that something of a plastic* nature is growing uncontrolledly? It means that the plastic* is working centrifugally, thus making the head large, and, in doing so, is no longer permitting the head to be permeated in the proper manner with imaginative forces. These must be supplied. Therefore one will let the child do consonantal eurythmy.

Here we have a question about "a two-year-old boy with a large head, who is nevertheless not hydrocephalic and is otherwise apparently healthy."

Here you have the effective antidote, in properly applied consonantal eurythmy. Here we have arrived at the point at which a thorough observation of the morphology, of the more profound morphological facts, can provide a direct indication for the eurythmic treatment.

Another: "a twelve and three-quarter-year-old boy whose growth in height is distinctly retarded, with no organic

* Rudolf Steiner uses in every case here the word "plastic".

findings other than worms; intelligent but intellectually quickly tired." A most interesting complex of symptoms, all of which indicate that the imaginative forces are insufficent, that the plastic forces in the organs are running rampant because of a lack of inner fictile forces, of plastic soul forces. These plastic forces of the soul are those which destroy parasites. It is no wonder that when these forces are insufficient the child has worms. Thus one should have him do consonantal eurythmy; therein lies the antidote. These associations will provide you with concrete indications of where you can employ eurythmy. Although the phenomena are somewhat camouflaged here, eurythmy will have an extraordinarily positive effect even in such cases, particularly if one complements it medicinally.

Here I have an interesting question that has been presented to me. Naturally I must answer the questions in principle. If complications of any sort should appear, they can later be taken into special consideration as the case demands. However, although it may be necessary to combine something else along with it, the matter has nevertheless been thoroughly dealt with from the side characterized.

"I have as a patient a five-year-old child who lost a great deal of blood as the result of a bullet wound suffered in the outbreaks of violence; two years ago a deformation of the joints set in. These are things which could lead to anaemia and similar conditions in adults. How could one help this child therapeutically?"

Here you have a deformation of the joints. That is an outwardly-working tendency of plastic forces that are unable to remain within. Thus these forces ray outwards, leaving the human being instead of working within him as they should. They will be reflected in the most effective manner precisely through the practice of consonantal eurythmy. In doing consonantal eurythmy you will call forth the objectively effective imaginations which offset the deformations. As the manner in which the question is placed quite correctly indicates, people in the future will in general tend to deform in the most manifold ways, because they will no longer be able to build up the normalizing human form out of the involuntarily active forces. Man will become free; he will gradually become free even in respect to the building up of his own form. However, he must then be able to do something with this freedom. He must go on to engender imaginations which continuously counter the deformation.

Now as to the other; you see that we are here concerned with a dearth of objective imagination. We could have to do with a deficiency of objective inspiration as well, which would express itself in a deformation of the rhythmic system, if I may call it that. In the case of a deformation of the rhythmic system, the objective inspiration which goes inwards does not encounter the circulatory rhythm in the proper manner. One can work towards a normalization of the situation by practising vowels in eurythmy. In eurythmy the vowels affect internal irregularities which are precisely not accompanied by morphological changes, even as consonantal eurythmy affects deformations and the tendency to deformation.

As I said earlier, it may nevertheless be necessary to render aid when something appears in particularly radical form, as in the case of the deformations of the joints that we just discussed. There it would be necessary to come to the assistance of the consonantal eurythmic process therapeutically. This consonantal process works by stimulating through its imagination the inner breathing of the organs orientated from without inwards and lying on the far side, of the intestinal wall: the lungs, the kidneys, the liver, and so on. When a person does consonantal eurythmy, it is a fact that particularly the back of the head, the lungs, the liver and the kidneys begin to sparkle and flash; something is really there that indicates the reaction of the spirit and soul to what is done outside in the consonants. Man becomes a shining being in these organs, and the movements that are carried out are in continuous opposition to the luminous movements within. In particular, there appears an entire luminous reproduction of the excretory process of the kidneys, through certain consonantal movements. One has a picture of the excretory process of the kidneys in this luminous process which comes about as the result of consonantal eurythmy. And that works over into the unconscious imagination. The whole process in which this part begins to shine is the same process that I described as being especially under the influence of copper. It is the same process. Here one must draw the attention of the physicians to the fact that there are people with particular forms of illness. These forms of illness were brought to my attention again yesterday when I was shown some painted pictures that were very much admired in some quarters at least, and was asked whether they were particularly occult. In a certain sense, of course, they are occult, but it is extraordinarily difficult to speak to people about these things, for they are an objectively-fixed kidney-efflorescence; they are the objectively-fixed process of the excretion of urine. When in the case of persons predisposed to this illness the process of urinary excretion becomes an abnormal, luminous process, that is, when the process of excretion falters — a purely metabolic illness — the kidneys then begin to shine. When this inwardly directed clairvoyance then sets in, people begin to draw wildly. What they produce will be aesthetic, in an outer formal manner beautiful in every case. The colours applied will be beautiful. But, of course, people are not content when one says to them, "Yes, there you have painted something very beautiful; it is in fact your obstructed excretion of urine." I can assure you that the obstructed urinary process and suppressed sexual desires — which lead as well in a certain manner to metabolic irregularities — are often presented by people of particularly mystical nature as mystically profound drawings and paintings. In much of what makes its appearance in the world in this manner one should recognize the symptoms of pathological abnormalities in the human being that are just bearable still.

As you see, anthroposophically oriented spiritual science is not mysticism as mysticism is commonly understood, since it fosters no illusions about matters such as we have just characterized. Quite the contrary: it investigates just such matters. People take exception to one for doing so, however. They resent my having gone so far in a public lecture as to indicate that the lovely poetry of Mechthild von Magdeburg, for example, or of Saint Theresa, are the inspirational reflexes of processes arising from repressed sexuality. Here, of course, the things are not drawn or painted, but poetically expressed. Naturally it is not pleasant for people to hear Mechthild von Magdeburg or Saint Theresa described as personalities with a strong sexuality which they restrained precisely because it was too strong for them, that certain metabolic-circulatory processes resulted from this retension, and that the reactions to this in turn appeared in such a form that they were fixed in very beautiful poetry. Indeed, this phenomenon leads extraordinarily deep into the mysteries of existence, when considered in a higher light. However, one must be able to rise to such an interpretation. And, therefore, one must have at least a notion of these peculiar processes which light up as inward processes when eurythmy is done outwardly. And in the moment when what is concealed within the poetry becomes eurythmy, as I showed you yesterday — when a beautiful poem is read and the eurythmy corresponding to it is done as we saw yesterday in vowels or consonants — then the one thing crosses the other; then an inward silent speaking joins what is carried out outwardly in movements in the person doing eurythmy as well. And when this process does not exude in sultry poetry but takes instead the course of accompanying beautiful poetry as eurythmy, then that which takes place in the human being does not become a recording of mysticism, but

86

a definite process of healing for the human being. Thus one can say that when one lets the patients do eurythmy in such a manner that one continually brings to his attention: listen carefully, bring intensely into consciousness the sound that you hear, the relationships of the sentence you hear, to which you are doing eurythmy; then one will initiate his ascent to the outward formative forces, to the objectively intuiting powers. When one wants to affect all that has remained in the human being from what no longer took place between birth and death, but what materialism calls inheritance — the greater part of which, however, is carried over from the pre-existent spiritual soul-life — if one wants to affect what can be called congenital defects and so on, then one will do well to work — particularly during the course of youth — again and again through eurythmy by challenging the person doing it: make very clear to yourself what you hear outwardly! By this method one can drive out all the tendencies to fix inwardly what would like to arise and take form in something like mystical poetry or mystical drawing. Precisely that will be connected to the beautiful outer poem. It is the reverse process. A true mystic knows that that of an abnormal nature which is reflected by the human being as beauty always has a questionable side. By contrast, one cannot claim that, when what is beautiful in the outer world is experienced inwardly, it appears as a particularly magnificent and beautiful picture: on the contrary, it becomes schematic and thereby abstract; abstract as if it were sketched; abstract, as a drawing is abstract. That is precisely what is healthy, however, and what is desired. The beautiful historic process would not have taken place, but if for example Mechthild von Magdeburg had been instigated to do eurythmy to good poetry, her entire mystic fate would have been spared her. Naturally one can say here that a point has been reached where in a certain sense good and evil cease to exist; one enters into the amoral sphere of Nietzsche, beyond good and evil. Of course, one cannot be so philistine as to claim that all the Mechthilds von Magdeburg should be eradicated. On the other hand you may be certain that from the supersensible worlds care will be taken that the corresponding connections with these supersensible worlds nevertheless remain, when man attempts to prevent this tendency from undue proliferation.

Although it is quite late, I would still like to go into a few matters in order to perhaps bring some clarification. I would like to start with the following question:

"Couldn't the therapeutic eurythmy exercises be reinforced by rational breathing exercises? It needn't necessarily be Hatha-Yoga."

To this I would like to make the following remark. In our times, and within the direction that the continually progressing human nature has taken, rational breathing exercises, as a reinforcement of the eurythmic exercises, can in fact only be treated in the following manner. It will be observed that a tendency towards a modification in the rhythm of respiration arises of its own accord under the influence of the vowels in eurythmy. One will notice this quite clearly. Here one finds oneself in the uncomfortable situation that one should avoid stereotyping, avoid saying the one thing or another in general, but should first observe what is to be done. One should concern oneself in each individual case with the breathing of the person in whose healing one is attempting to be of assistance by means of eurythmic vowel exercises (in accordance with the diagnosis given, whatever it may be); one should observe the modification of the breathing and subsequently make the patient aware that he can consciously pursue this tendency himself. We are no longer human beings like the ancient orientals, who would go the reverse route and influence the entire human being by way of a prescribed method of breathing. This is something which today leads of necessity, in every case, to inner shocks, no matter how it is prescribed; it should really be avoided. We just have to learn to notice what kind of effect eurythmy itself, especially vocalic eurythmy, has on the breathing process. And then we can consciously continue the tendency which arises eurythmically, in the individual case. You will certainly observe that this respiratory process will be carried on individually, continued in varying manners in different people.

My esteemed friends, those are more or less the things that it is possible to answer at the moment. We have no real possibility of dealing with a number of matters that have got bogged down due to the shortness of time. In closing, my dear friends. I want to warn you that you must be prepared that your medical colleagues in the world will wage their wars no less intensely when they become aware of your bringing something of our sort to bear, and that you will have need of the penetrating power of conviction to weaken what will confront you. In no case, of course, may what you are confronted with lead you to neglect these matters; we may permit ourselves no illusions about those antagonistic forces we arouse.

At the end of this course I would as well like to state that, in order to make the movement possible, as it should now be inaugurated in the medical field, I will adhere everywhere to the policy of not involving myself directly with the patients in the therapeutic process, but will discuss and consult only with the physicians themselves. Thus you will always be in the position to refute any allegations that I myself interfere in any way in an unjustified manner in the therapy. I have already mentioned this at the end of the last course. This has been made extraordinarily difficult for me even from the anthroposophical side — this cannot be passed over in silence — as people naturally make all possible demands in this direction. It is also definitely the case that among anthroposophists the tendency exists, not only *not* to rise above egoism, but sometimes to become even more egoistic than normal people are. Then, when the occasion arises it is often a matter of complete indifference to the person, what the welfare of the movement may entail; that the welfare of the movement is dependent in each individual instance upon a rejection of the practice of what the world outside terms quackery; that a healing process should take place in the whole of medicine and should not be disturbed by the demands arising from an individual's personal aspirations. People will make it difficult, but it must be carried through in this direction, since we will only be able to succeed in this area when we can stand up to the outer world — as we are otherwise able to, in the anthroposophical movement, insofar as matters are conducted with understanding and not bowdlerized by people without understanding. Simply by virtue of knowing what is going on in the anthroposophical movement we must be in the position to say: what is being said there is certainly a lie, it is beyond doubt an invention. We must simply always be in the position to say that, in certain cases. And we come to be able to say that, when we are all inwardly initiated in the contents of matters such as those to which I have drawn attention here: that I myself do not intervene in the therapeutic process, but that within the anthroposophical movement the doctors are responsible for the therapy of the patients.

Having said what was necessary, I want to add nothing more than the wish that the stimuli — which, in this course in particular, have often remained mere indications — may work on in you and become active in the appropriate manner for the welfare of humanity. Hopefully we will have the opportunity to carry on in some manner what we have already twice begun; in any case we will make an effort to carry on with it. With this wish, my dear friends, I will close these contemplations, in the hope that our deeds in these directions may be in accord with our wishes. It was very satisfying to see you here. It will be a satisfying feeling to think back on these days here, which it was your desire to spend together towards the enrichment of medical science. The thoughts that hold us together will accompany you, my dear friends, on the paths that you will wander, to transform into deeds what we attempted to activate, to begin with here, as thoughts.

LECTURE 8

Stuttgart, October 28, 1922   (held before physicians)

The wish has been expressed for me to expound somewhat further upon curative eurythmy. Basically, the empiric material related to curative eurythmy was developed and presented in the last course for physicians in Dornach, and it is hardly necessary to go beyond what was given at that time. Used in the proper manner, it will be of far-reaching importance. Today I would like to speak to you about the whole purpose and meaning of curative eurythmy.

Curative eurythmy took shape out of something purely artistic, out of what was first developed as an artistic impulse; and in certain connections a basis for the correct understanding of curative eurythmy must be taken from artistic eurythmy. Now perhaps I will be most clearly understood if at first I attempt to indicate the difference between artistic and curative eurythmy. Eurythmy in general is based on the possibility of transforming in a certain direction what takes place in the human organism in speech. For this reason eurythmy is, artistically, really a sort of visible speech. We must recognize that two components work together in human speech. One component originates through a particular use of the formative apparatus — of which I may speak on the basis of the preceding lectures — from a layer of the nervous system which lies further inward. What is related to the mental image plays in here. Esentially the apparatus of mental representation in the speech apparatus extends itself, to be sure in a somewhat complicated way, even into the construction of the nervous system, and it is exactly this which then produces in the further radiation one of the components at work in speech. The other component comes up out of the human being's metabolism. In a way we have a meeting of two dynamic systems, one coming out of the human metabolism and another arising from the nerve-sensory system. The two encounter each other in such a way that the metabolic system is transformed first into the circulatory processes; and that which has to do with mental representation, coming from the nerve-sensory system is metamorphosed into the respiratory system. In the respiratory and circulatory systems these two dynamic systems converge, and, since the whole is carried over into the air by means of the speech-system, it is possible for the human astral organism to stream into what is created there as movement of air. If we consider the outermost periphery of the human organism, we see that speech comes into being through an embodiment on the one hand of what has to do with mental picturing and on the other, of the metabolic nature which, when expressed in terms of the soul, is actually the will-nature. Thus we have what finds its expression in the soul as will, and bodily its expression in the metabolic system, that is, to the extent in which the nervous system has a part in the will (which it in fact has, insofar as metabolism takes place — not as nerve-sensory activity — in the nervous system). Thus, what is of a volitional nature and finds its bodily expression in the metabolic system, and that which is of the nature of mental representation which finds its expression in what I would like to call a section or stratum of the nerve-sensory system, conjoin to form what results. They then find physical expression in what manifests as ordinary speech or singing. In the case of song it is something different but nonetheless similar. In eurythmy one blocks out what is of the nature of mental representation to the greatest possible degree and brings volition into force. In this way ordinary speech is metamorphosed into movements of the entire human organism: one strengthens one component, the will or the metabolism, one weakens the mental representation or the nerve-sensory, and one has as a result eurythmy. In this way one is really in the position to create correlatives in human movement for the individual sounds, whether they be vowels or consonants. Just as a certain formation and movement of air can correspond to an A or an L, so can an outwardly visible form in movement correspond to an A or an L. Here we have a movement, or movement structure, as I would like to call it, derived from the human organism through sensible-supersensible vision; which proceeds from the human organism with the same lawfulness as speech in sounds and which, although more volitionally-oriented, is only a meta-morphosis of this speech. One can compose the entire alphabet in this speech; one can bring everything linguistic to expression through this eurythmy. When artistic eurythmy is performed, the attention of the human being and all the processes in the human physical, etheric and astral organisms which mediate this alertfulness, are directed to the corresponding sound, to the formation of the word or the artistic formation of the sentence, to the metric form, the poetic form and so on. When active in artistic eurythmy, one is completely absorbed in the possibilities of artistic formation and portrayal of the elements of speech. The human being surrenders to the outer world when he is artistically active in eurythmy, since in eurythmy one naturally follows the structure ("Gestaltüng") that is also common to speech. And since one does not stop at an A or an L in the middle of a word, but carries on further, in artistic eurythmy we have to do with something that may quite possibly take place in the normally functioning human organism. Ordinary artistic eurythmy has no other physiological consequences for the human organism other than that this artistic eurythmy calls forth in an energetic manner an inner harmony in the human functions, insofar as these functions form a totality in the human organism.

Thus one can say that when one refrains in the right manner from exaggeration in eurythmic artistic activity, it is conducive to health. But just as everything conducive to health can also make one sick if exaggerated, the artistic practice of eurythmy can be overdone. Professor Benedikt, the famous criminal psychologist, emphasized repeatedly — because he could not endure the anti-alcohol movement — that more people die from water than from alcohol. Even the statistics must concede this: over-indulgence in water leads to numerous sorts of illness. Eurythmy, in general, as long as it remains within the appropriate limits, can only be conducive to health; a certain artistic feeling of satisfaction or dissatisfaction will arise in any case.

That which lives in the devotion to the sound- word- and sentence-formation in artistic eurythmy is reflected inwards in curative eurythmy. It is reflected inwards simply through the fact that in curative eurythmy the sound A, for example, must be repeated a number of times in succession. By this means, something entirely different is achieved than when I pass over from the sound A to an I or something else in an artistic presentation. Now it will be a question of gaining insight into the actual therapeutic process which can take place through eurythmy. I cannot avoid expressing concern about something which lies close at hand here: amateurs and dilettants appropriate such things very easily. From the beginning I have emphasized that curative eurythmy should be practised by the doctor himself or herself, or at the very least should only be practised in the most intimate coll-aboration with a doctor. The attitude which spiritual science takes in relation to such offshoots will be taken as indicative of spiritual science's position in regard to medicine as a whole.

Spiritual science does not operate in the field of medicine in such a manner as I once encountered twenty years ago. People who called themselves nature-therapy doctors were present at an anthroposophical convention and presented me with a treatise in which it was repeatedly stated in a variety of ways: all healing is based upon bringing into harmony what is inharmonious in the organism. This sentence was repeated for six pages in the most manifold variations: one should harmonize the disharmonious. There is nothing at all that one can object to in this sentence, it is only that one must be able to do it in a specific manner in a particular case. That is where it becomes unpleasant for people who hold an opinion such as was expressed in their final sentence: everything which has been said above proves that one can leave the unbelievably complicated medicine behind and restrict oneself to harmonizing the disharmonious. That would be, in their own words, "intoxicatingly simple." Something so intoxicatingly simple I can't offer you. Medicine cannot be driven into intoxicating simplicity by spiritual science, but rather to greater complexity, as you will have gathered by now from various instances. Through spiritual science you will not have less to learn, but more, but there is a snag attached to learning less anyway, because through learning more everything will become clearer and more ordered and the learning thereby more interesting. Whoever had the idea that healing would be made easier through spiritual science will already have been convinced by the expositions that I have made here that this is not the case.

And so it is with curative eurythmy. It is definitely the case that curative eurythmy should not be applied without a thorough diagnosis and that it should only be practised in agreement with professional medical science, for the reason that one has to do here with the application of an exceedingly intimate knowledge of the human organism.

Because of the fact that in normal speech the metabolic activity and the plastic activity of the nerve-sensory system collide with one another, the result of this collision, is unloaded in the movement of the air (This is something which takes place in relative isolation from the human organism so that as a result speech is released from the organism.) all of what is shaped through curative eurythmy is thrown back into the organism, and one has thus to do with the following. Imagine that you place an A-movement together with an L-movement. First of all you have the movements repeated, so that the whole affair is not discharged outside, but rather that the repetition pours into the inner processes of the human organism. By allowing the vowel and consonantal elements, let us say in the A-movement and the L-movement, to work together, you will always induce a functioning in the human organism that implies a mutual activity of the metabolic-man and the nerve-sensory-man. To be sure, the activity of the nerve-sensory system is in any case weakened in eurythmy, but the two components, the dampened nerve-sensory activity and the heightened metabolic activity brought about by the eurythmic movement, work together in this exceptional proportion nevertheless. One has simply, a driving of the metabolic-man against the nerve-sensory-man, when one does the L-movement repeatedly, and when the L-movement is associated with an A-form. Thus one can say: the entire functioning of the human organism is carried along with the instigation of the forms and movements necessary. When, for example, you let someone carry out a consonantal movement, it works, to begin with, in such a way that it in essence unloads its whole power, its inner dynamic, on the process of inhalation; the whole procedure of inhalation actually lies in your control. According to the consonants you induce, you have the entire process of in-breathing in your hands. You strengthen the process of inhalation through each consonantal activity.

You perhaps know, from what has already been told about curative eurythmy, that movements of artistic eurythmy are somewhat modified for curative eurythmy. One can say that when an A- or an L-movement is carried out, it is always associated with a strengthening or weakening of the thrust initiated by inhalation. You must take inhalation into consideration here in its entirety. In examining the in-breath, we must to begin with follow its path into the middle part of the human organism, and then, however, through the medial canal, vertebral ("Rückenmarkscanal") canal into the brain. The activity of the brain is in essence the harmonising of the breathing activity, in its refinement within the brain, with the nerve-sensory activity. There is no activity of the brain which may be considered alone; every such activity results from the nerve-sensory activity and the breathing activity. All the activities of the brain must be studied in such a way that respiration is taken into consideration. By inducing certain consonants, various consonants, you can, by way of the breath, influence the plastic activity of man, the sculptural activity, in the most striking manner. In the case of a child who is getting his second teeth, for example, you have only to know from a certain artistic grasp of the human organism how the upper teeth will be built up out of plastic activity which works from above downwards. In the case of the upper teeth, the plastic activity that forms them is active from the front backwards. How will the lower teeth be formed? In the teeth of the lower jaw the plastic activity works from the back to the front. If I were to express schematically the activity going on in teething, it would be as follows: the upper teeth are built up from front to back; thus, the back surfaces are shaped and the front surfaces are deposited. The lower teeth are built up from back to front. This is the manner in which the forces work together.

If you notice that a child is having difficulties in teething, you can assist the process in the maxilla, for example, simply by having the child do the movement for A. You can support the same process in the lower jaw with the O-movement. You can in fact gain control over the fictile powers through specific instigation. In order to give this plastic activity nourishment, so to speak, you must direct your attention principally to supporting the thrust that accompanies the inhalation; you must add to the plastic activity accomplished in this way by the A- and O-movements what you observe resulting from the entire human constitution. Let us say we have a person with weak peristalsis, who is somewhat inclined to constipation. In the period of life in which teething takes place, the intestinal activity is related to the building up of the teeth, and one must focus one's attention there, where irregularities in teething have their origin. If you wish to come to the assistance of the thrust of breath which travels through the vertebral canal into the brain and expedites from there the formative forces, which one has in one's power through the movements for vowels, you will be able to do this, if you have precisely such a case before you by having the child carry out the movmeent for L. If you simply study curative eurythmy, the way in which you should apply it will become clear to you through the diagnosis. Without a diagnosis it should not be practised, because in certain circumstances one can do entirely the wrong thing. However, it is indeed a fact that one must awaken in oneself a feeling for the artistic in the dynamics of the human being as a whole. One must develop an intuitive glance for the artistic. Let us assume that the child is observed to have certain difficulties at the time it begins to teethe; it has certain disorders which shouldn't be present. One discovers that the intestinal movement is irregular and insufficient. With the L-movement one is properly prepared. After one has done the L-movement for a time, one comes to the assistance of what one has conducted to the formative centre with the movement for A or O. The vowel movements affect the exhalation and begin to work already in the brain. The stream of breath works in the brain. Everything associated with inhalation, in its most extensive, inclusive sense, expresses itself in the consonantal element. That can be reinforced and promoted through consonantal eurythmy. Everything having to do with exhalation can be reinforced by doing the vowels in eurythmy. When you do the vowels in eurythmy, the plastic element works directly together with the radiating element. You must judge, by how much strength must be applied, how many times the sound must be repeated. Let us say, for example, we have to do with a kidney disturbance of one sort or another. You may say to yourself that the kidney disturbance is in one stage or another, let us say in the beginning stage. The moment that I have certain movements performed — S-movements, for example* — I will have a beneficial effect on the kidney disturbance in its early stages. If the kidney distrubance has been present a considerable length of time, and the insufficient function has led already to deformation, I must then first prepare the ground with consonantal eurythmy and follow with the vowels; in order to work on formation through the vowels as opposed to the deformation which has already taken place. In short, one must approach the matter as untheoretically as possible; one must discover, solely out of knowledge of the human organism in its healthy and diseased states, what was given in the rules I set out in Dornach that have been passed on to you.

Now if, for example, it should be a case of suppressed heart-lung function which in turn affects the kidneys, one will make progress in the beginning stages with the movement for B or P. From this you will see that one has the entire functioning within one's grasp here, and that everything depends upon one's understanding that a sort of centrifugal dynamic is present in each separate human organ which is rounded-off plastically by another dynamic working from without inwards — a dynamic which is not exactly centripetal, but which could be designated as a similar-to-centripetal dynamic that works into every human organ. One will only be able to pursue the study of physiology properly when one is able to contemplate each separate human organ in its polarity. These polarities lie within, a centrifugal and a centripetal, in each human organ. For everything that is of a sculptural nature, the distribution and differentiation of the relative warmth and the organization of the air-conditions play a great role. For everything which is centrifugal, radiating, a great role is played by what in the human organism comes from the dynamic of the substances of the world themselves

* In another transcript A appears here rather than S. —German editor.

and what is developed in surmounting the vitality proper to external nature ("der äusseren Wesenheit") in the human organism. These two dynamics must be regulated reciprocally, and one can hope that curative eurythmists come forth who will cultivate a fine feeling for what can be achieved in different instances. Precisely here will extraordinarily much depend upon the artistic disposition of the soul.

Now when you take into consideration that the whole system of curative eurythmy can be reinforced by actual therapeutic methods, you find you have two factors which work together. One can say to oneself, such and such affects the heart in particular in this or that way; one can reinforce that effect with a curative eurythmy exercise: then one thing will promote the other in a complementary manner. That is something which opens up truly great vistas, which can have an extraordinarily great future. Just think of the effect of massage, in some instances. I do not want to say anything against it or to criticise it; I acknowledge its importance. Yet this outward scratching about on the human being is inconsequential in comparison to the massage that you apply when you induce entire systems of organs which work together to move inwardly in a different manner, through the elements of curative eurythmy. That is the most inward kneading of the whole organism, linked with effects in the etheric, the astral, the ego organisms. Thus it is possible to say that what one recognizes as correct in massage is, in an unendingly powerful way, made inward through curative eurythmy. One will in fact first gain an insight into the curative effects of gymnastics as well when one examines the resemblance between gymnastic exercises and eurythmic exercises. What is therapeutic in gymnastics is only of secondary importance to what is of significance in curative eurythmy. As I said at that time in Dornach, if one has the E-movement carried out in a rhythmic sequence in the manner that was then demonstrated, one does a great deal to help weak-looking children — children who only feebly carry through their bodily functions — to become healthier and to begin to become stronger, as one would wish to see them. It is, however, necessary that one takes the whole human being into consideration in such matters. Again and again it happens that the entire human being is taken too little into consideration. I know that that is a triviality, for you will say: "We know that, of course." Indeed, but again and again in practice it is not taken into consideration. How often one hears: this person has an irregularly functioning heart, something must be done for it. Yes, but if one were to take the total human being into consideration one would have to say: thank God that he has such a heart; his organism couldn't tolerate a normal one. Similarly, for example, under certain circumstances one would have to say of a person who had broken his nose, that he had suffered a favourable stroke of fate: if he breathed in air through completely developed channels, he would have too much air for his organism to process. What has its foundations in the organism as a whole must everywhere be taken into consideration.

When the movements for "I" are carried out in a certain manner, they tend to harmonize the association of the right and the left sides of the human organism. With "I" one can be of help in all asymmetries that appear in the human organism. Through the cautious use of "I"-movements one can have excellent results with curative eurythmy, even in the case of squinting. With squinting I would only advise that one does not proceed as one would with a person who walks asymmetrically, for example, or who can use the right and left arms too asymmetrically. For squinting I would apply the usual I-movements but would carry them out only with the index finger, and in this way I would have them repeated as often as possible during the day. When the person is still growing this can bring good results, especially if the "I" is carried out with the big toe as well. The best results will be achieved, however, when one can bring the patient to do it

101

with the little toe as well. On the asymmetries affecting the sight these eurythmic exercises performed at the periphery will have a most beneficial effect. On the other hand, when it is a question of evening-out an indexterity in the manner in which a person walks, it could even bring good results to have him do the reverse: that is, to carry out the I-movement with the line of vision, as when sighting. Provided, of course, it does him no harm. In fact, one can really establish a sort of law: everything which is abnormal in the lower human being tends to be normalized by what is created as a compensation in the upper man, and vice versa.

When you find insecurities in standing, which may, of course, arise in the most varied manners, the forms of "U" will be of especial importance. However, you must see that the U-form is brought to completion so that the limbs concerned are really contiguous. This being in direct contact with one another, so that one limb feels the other, is of particular importance. Only then is the U-form complete. In artistic eurythmy it is only necessary to indicate that this is so; in curative eurythmy, however, it must be carried out: one limb is brought up against the other so that one stands as when "at attention" — with the legs pressed against one another. That is an extraordinarily curative exercise for people who are affected with a compulsive twitching in the head. When it is fitting to treat corpulent children by means of curative eurythmy, the O-forms serve the purpose well. All these forms, however, if they are intended to bring results as curative eurythmy, must be combined with a distinct perception of the muscle system involved. If you simply make the O-form as many eurythmists do, it will suffice as an outward indication. It will not have a curative effect, however, unless in the process of doing the exercise you feel the muscles throughout the arm. The slack swinging form has no effect; the sensation of the whole muscle system in its details, however, will bring the respective curative eurythmic result. It is particularly important to take heed that the curative eurythmic exercise is strengthened by extending it into the consciousness. When you do the O-movement as I just did it, it is associated with a strong projection into the consciousness. Tell the obese person whom you treat with the O-form: "think of your obesity, of your own girth, when doing the 'O'!" In this way the consciousness centres on exactly that which is to be remedied. You thereby reinforce in its innermost nature what is intended, namely, that the element of consciousness is not in the least to be underestimated in healing.

In this connection I have reason to believe that when these things become known, a battle with the orthopedists will take place. Despite the fact that they are experiencing a great deal of success in their field at the present time, they are quite intent on treating the human being as a sort of mechanism. In the case of appliances used therapeutically in such a way that the person in question should continually feel them, that they enter his awareness, this consciousness is an excellent curative factor. Let us say, for example, that I find it would be advantageous for someone to straighten his shoulders; and I give him bandages which bring to his awareness that the shoulders should be held back — in other words, so that the treatment isn't carried out unconsciously. It is exactly the same in curative eurythmy: these matters are brought to consciousness, in order that, as I have already said, this concentration vitally reinforce the curative eurythmic element itself.

Let us go on to something of particular importance which I want to tell you. Everything that is an E-form has a regulatory effect where the astral organism affects the etheric organism either too strongly or too weakly. Thus in all those cases where one determines that either an exaggerated or an insufficient activity of the astral organism is present, one will under circumstances be able to achieve a great deal with the E-forms, with the repetition of the E-forms. E-forms could have a curative effect upon both complexes of symptoms which I described in the previous hour. What I have just said is particularly true when the astral organism is under the influence of the etheric, when it is too weak, when it permits itself to be influenced by the etheric, which itself is too strong as the result of an irregularity in the astral organism of the head. The opposite condition in which the etheric is too strongly affected by the astral may also arise. That would be the case when the astral comes very forcefully to expression in the intestine: when one gets diarrhoea on every occasion when one is a bit afraid. The U-forms will have an especially advantageous effect here.

Yesterday a question arose which I would like to discuss briefly here, in closing: can one allow persons who are pregnant or who have gynaecological complaints to do certain eurythmic movements? Just examine what was given as a rule in Dornach. You should be able to adhere to it even though in the case of pregnant women and gynaecological patients you must make certain that the abdomen is left in peace. It must be left undisturbed. it must not be irritated by curative eurythmic exercises. Although the abdomen itself is left in peace, exercises may nevertheless definitely be done with the arms while sitting, or while lying down, with the head; and while that which must have quiet is in complete repose. You will still find enough in the indications given to be able to take measures through curative eurythmy. Naturally when the person cannot move at all, eurythmy would be quite the most beneficial for him, as in the case of paralytic symptoms; but under the circumstances the person cannot carry them out. They would definitely be the most wholesome. Such paralytic symptoms are of course in essence an abnormal functioning of the astral body, which does not engage itself in the etheric and physical organisation. Here one will be able to achieve a great deal with E-movements. An E-movement that is very beneficial for disturbances of the abdomen is the carefully performed, not exaggerated, artificial crossing of the eyes. It is in fact true that the somewhat decadent yogis who do certain exercises in which they focus their eyes on the tip of the nose, really intend to evoke the most harmonic activity of the abdomen possible, since they know the significance of abdominal activity for what such people call spiritual activity. Thus one can say: matters are such that one can simply replace, with a lighter eurythmy of the arms, the fingers, or even the eyes when it is necessary, certain things that a person with a healthy abdomen would do with jumps. A pregnant woman should never be induced to do curative eurythmy exercises with jumps. That, of course, won't do.

As you see, it was not intended to produce a panacea that could be learnt in half a day. Curative eurythmy too must be acquired through earnest labour, and it is necessary in fact that it is acquired through practice. For practically every time you put the curative eurythmy exercises into practice, with the help of your curative exercises, you will be able to make better use of them. It is indeed so: through practice one will make exceptionally good progress, most particularly in curative eurythmy.

Now it was my intention to present you with this more theoretical discussion of curative eurythmy, because everything else having to do with it, to the extent curative eurythmy exists today, was given earlier in Dornach and will be handed on by our physician friends and thus be available to you; and because I wanted to give you the possibility of understanding the whole physiological and therapeutic meaning of eurythmy. Of course, on the other hand, one must not overestimate something like curative eurythmy. In many cases it will be an extraordinarily important resource, but one should not overestimate it. One must make clear to oneself that really nothing can be achieved with intoxicating simplicity; one can no more heal a broken leg or broken arm through curative exercises alone, than one can heal a carcinoma through the intoxicating simplicity of harmonizing the disharmonious. One must be entirely clear that it is not an increase in dilettantism and medical amateurism which is to be found on the path of spiritual science, but rather a definite enrichment of professional medical ability. Excuse me for emphasizing it so often; in order to prevent misunderstandings, however, I particularly want to stress again that the methods are not brought forward in amateurish opposition to official medicine, as is often the case in fanatical movements. They take into account the state of medical science at present, and desire only to lead it along the path along which it must be led, for the simple reason that it is not true that the human being is only that which the physiology and anatomy of today maintain he is. He is that, to be sure, but he is something more as well: he must be recognized from the aspect of his soul and spirit. Then those peculiar mental pictures that constantly show up nowadays, in which the brain for example is seen as a sort of central telegraphic apparatus to which the so-called sensory nerves run, and from which the motor nerves lead, will disappear. The whole matter has no relation to reality, as will have become clear to you through today's lecture. In the nerve-sensory system one has rather to do with a sort of modelling dynamic, from which something is wrung which then accommodates itself to the activity of the soul. There is a great deal to be done in order to give back to a healthy physiology what has been taken from it through the correlations incorrectly established between the physical organism and the functions of the soul. Something physical is indeed present for every function of the soul during the course of man's life on earth, but, on the other hand, nothing is used for the soul which has not a much greater importance for the bodily organization in its reciprocal action with the other organs. Nothing which is used for the soul is used merely as an organ of the soul. Our entire soul and spiritual make-up is wrested from the bodily nature, is taken out of the bodily. We may not permit ourselves to indicate certain organs as belonging to the soul. We could only say that the

106

soul-functions are such that they are disengaged from the organic functions and are particularly adapted to the activity of the soul. Only when we become earnest about what is at work in the human organism, when we no longer proceed in so outward a fashion, that we picture the whole nervous system as an insertion serving the life of the soul can we hope to perceive the human organization as it is. Only when the human organism is so perceived can it provide the basis for a physiology and therapy which work in the light, not grope in the dark. I make this last remark to you, so that you yourselves do not leave here under a misunderstanding, and to enable you to counter misunderstandings which arise again and again.

Our carcinoma medication, for example, has been criticized with the "intoxicating simplicity" that arises from having no idea whatever about the knowledge through which one has arrived at the medication. People have constructed instead some simple analogy or another and believe that in disposing of the analogy, one can have done with the matter itself. A proviso for the development and growth of the spiritual-scientific side of medicine is that one confront the misunderstandings at least to a degree. People will soon notice that when they cannot spread misunderstandings, they will have very little at all to say, for the principal concern of the opponents is the broadcasting of misconceptions about the whole of Anthroposophy. Count how many adversaries have something other than misconceptions to relate. I must say that I often read antagonistic articles or essays and could connect them with something else entirely, were my name not present. It has no relation to what is nurtured here; it deals with something entirely different. Sometimes I am very much surprised and would like to go and search out where that which is being refuted has been expounded; in any case not here. In medicine the same thing is done as in theology; there one encounters it as well. One can, for example, say to a theologian at the pinnacle of science: we have the same to say about the Christ as you, only somewhat more. He is, however, not content when one says what he himself says, and then something in addition. He maintains one should not add anything to it. He does not criticize what is contrary to his assertions, he criticizes what he says nothing at all about. He criticizes what is said, simply because one speaks about something he knows nothing about. He considers it a mistake to know something about what he knows nothing about. Medicine must not fall into this error. We must observe accurately, and, rather than contradicting, we must *add* a great deal, out of an extremely well-founded knowledge of the healthy and diseased human being.

References to books related to passages in the text

Page 2 "...metamorphic variation... Goetheanistic contemplation..." see: *Goethes Naturwissenschaftliche Schriften*, edited by Rudolf Steiner, Kurschner's "Deutsche National-Literature", Vol. 1, Troxler-Verlag Bern 1949

Page 65 The lecture which appears here as number seven (April 18, 1921) was given in connection with the so-called second course for physicians and is printed in the book *Geisteswissenschaftliche Gesichtspunkte zur Therapie*, Dornach 1963, as well. Rudolf Steiner refers to this lecture at the end of the foregoing with the words: "After a short pause we will proceed with greater reference to eurythmy."

Page 79 The eighth lecture was given in connection with the "Medical Week" held in Stuttgart from the 26th to the 28th of October 1922 (see *Physiologisch-Therapeutisches auf Grundlage der Geisteswissenschaft*, Dornach 1965.) This lecture is printed only here.

Page 92 "E-forms could have a curative effect upon both complexes of symptoms which I described in the previous hour." See the fourth lecture in the series: *Anthroposophische Grundlagen für die Arzneikunst*, in *Physiologisch-Therapeutisches auf Grundlage der Geisteswissenschaft*. Dornach 1965, page 140

COMMENTS BY THE EDITOR

OF THE THIRD GERMAN EDITION

The present edition of this course — which Rudolf Steiner gave in 1921 in order to bring to realization the hygienic-therapeutic side of eurythmy, which, as he explained in his introductory words to eurythmy performances, was given this name to distinguish it from artistic and pedagogical eurythmy — is the first edition to appear in print and be available to a wider public. Since those days curative eurythmy has become much used on a worldwide scale as a therapy in connection with medicine, and it takes its place alongside other recognized therapies in the same way as, according to Rudolf Steiner, artistic eurythmy does among the other arts.

In the main there are two things to be said about this edition. Firstly, — and Rudolf Steiner said this very strongly — curative eurythmy must only be given when a doctor prescribes it and is in charge of it. Secondly, a proper training in eurythmy is required as a preliminary to learning curative eurythmy for use as a therapy. Rudolf Steiner said that at least two years should be spent on a thorough study of eurythmy. The normal eurythmy training takes four years at present. As this course is now available to everyone, it should be said that it is quite impossible to study curative eurythmy on one's own with the help of this book. Collaboration with a doctor and the study of eurythmy are both inescapable. Rudolf Steiner puts it in the following way in the "Course for Curative Education" (Rudolf Steiner Press, 1981)

"When you bring curative eurythmy into curative education you are bringing the whole of eurythmy into it. So you

109

should be aware that you must acquire a living connection with it, and this should be such that anyone who does curative eurythmy ought to a certain point to have learnt basic eurythmy. Curative eurythmy ought to be based on a general knowledge of speech and tone eurythmy, even if artistic perfection has not been attained. Then, above all, people must be filled with the conviction that they must work with others, and therefore, when curative eurythmy is going to be put into practice the therapist must get the support of a doctor. When curative eurythmy was given to the world it was stipulated that it should not be put into practice without the collaboration of a doctor. All this points to how inter-connected in a living way, things have to be when they come out of Anthroposophy."

The present lectures — with the exception of the one given on April 18, — were made available in manuscript form by Frau Marie Steiner in 1930. They were edited by Elisabeth Baumann, who had taken part in the course. Rudolf Steiner's executors produced a new edition in 1952 edited by I. de Jaager. The lecture to doctors given on October 28, 1922 was included in this edition. Both these editors made important comments on the course and summaries of these will follow.

For the present edition the notes were examined and the whole text checked against the available shorthand reports. Some additions and corrections could consequently be made. Some parts that had been revised now follow the shorthand notes more closely.

Where the story of eurythmy is concerned a detailed account is given in the volume of Rudolf Steiner's complete works "Die Entstehung und Entwickelung der Eurythmie" (the origins and development of eurythmy).

The following words are taken from Frau Baumann's introduction: "Children of all ages grasped and carried out the movements of eurythmy so naturally that we experienced every day of our lives that the visible language of eurythmy movement is a language that is in genuine harmony with the laws and requirements of both man's spiritual-soul nature and his bodily nature. We also experienced daily that hindrances the children had, whether in the realm of the will or in the realm of thought — the thinking activity — could be loosened up or actually overcome by eurythmy. At the Waldorf School we had to deal with children, almost from the very beginning, who had hindrances of this sort. Sometimes these difficulties were only slightly in evidence, sometimes the children were so overwhelmed by them, that they could not keep up with the lessons of their class, and a special remedial class was started where they could be given what Rudolf Steiner prescribed for their care.

Experience showed that for children of this sort eurythmy more than anything else could get across to them and they could take immediate hold of it. Therefore we asked ourselves whether it would be possible to find exercises that would help the spiritual part that was having such difficulty in incarnating because it met with such strong bodily resistance — exercises that would give the physical sheath a better form, movement exercises which would help the etheric formative forces to penetrate better and give their support to the creative upbuilding forces of the organism.

Out of our close connection with so-called difficult cases, with retarded children, with those in need of special care, we acquired the most intense desire to discover and take hold of the hygienic, curative element of eurythmy. From many conversations with Erna van Deventer-Wolfram, who was actively engaged in eurythmy in various parts of Germany, it transpired that through the work she was doing she, too, had been powerfully drawn to this curative aspect of eurythmy. After due reflection we decided to ask Dr. Steiner for instructions on curative eurythmy. Rudolf Steiner agreed with alacrity and promised to think about it. It was not long before Frau van Deventer and I were requested to go to Dornach in April where he wanted to give lectures on curative eurythmy alongside the doctors' course he was

111

going to give at the Goetheanum.

And so during the days of April 12 to 17, 1921, Rudolf Steiner presented the gift of the third element of eurythmy, and the doctors and eurythmists who were present experienced a whole new world of possibilities for therapy opening up before them, which, in its variety and effectiveness and the way in which Rudolf Steiner presented it, is bound to have made an unforgettable impression on them. Instead of the few instructions and indications we had asked for we were given a complete and detailed method of eurythmy therapy in which we could directly experience that even today the creative and curative power of the Word, with its capacity to take hold of the movement potential in the human body, is still at work. It often happened that it was not easy to find our way into it, for even those of us who had been familiar with the eurythmic art of movement for many years found that the exercises Rudolf Steiner either performed himself or asked Frau van Deventer-Wolfram and myself to perform were utterly new and surprising. It was especially difficult for the doctors present, as only a minority had had anything to do with eurythmy up till then. Two eurythmy courses were organized where we discussed and practised basic eurythmy with the doctors, and also the exercises that had been given by Dr. Steiner in the curative eurythmy lecture that day.

Regular work at curative eurythmy now started up in various places. In the clinics in Arlesheim and Stuttgart and also at the Waldorf School, Rudolf Steiner gave several more indications for the use of curative eurythmy in special cases, he himself varied one or another exercise, and he gave certain sound sequences that were to be practised with individual patients under his special observation. These indications offer doctors and curative eurythmists a rich opportunity to learn more about a methodical approach, adapting of exercises to the individual needs of patients, and the scrupulous observation required for this.

The real basis of all curative eurythmy work is given in this course, as is clearly stated in Rudolf Steiner's own words. In October 1922, on the occasion of a medical week in Stuttgart he was again asked to speak about curative eurythmy, this time by doctors. That lecture is included here with the 1921 course. Right at the beginning Rudolf Steiner says "I have been requested to say something more about this curative eurythmy of ours. Fundamentally speaking I presented the empirical material for this curative eurythmy at the last doctors' course in Dornach (see "The Spiritual Scientific Aspect of Therapy"), and it is hardly necessary to go further than that. For if it is put to proper use it can have far-reaching significance."

From Frau I. de Jaager's epilogue (1952 edition):

"It will soon be evident to the reader that unless you make a thorough study of Anthroposophy you will not get very far with this curative eurythmy course. Curative eurythmy arises out of Anthroposophy just the same as artistic eurythmy does. A living grasp of Man and the world is a necessary basis for its use. Only on this assumption will it avoid becoming a system or something that is grasped and applied in an abstract, intellectual way; a danger that is ever present in our times. Curative eurythmy also requires an extensive knowledge of artistic eurythmy. Imaginative forces, the coming into motion of the whole being of man, are prerequisites for the application of this therapy, where it is essential to have an artistic understanding of the patient. All the delicate and minute nuances we need in order to help a sick child or adult come to us out of artistic eurythmy. You will continually find new inspiration there.

I would like to stress that a young person should not devote herself exclusively to curative eurythmy. Up to the age of 28 a person should be able to give her imagination

113

and creative forces free rein. The more this can happen the better she will be able to develop devotion, patience and empathy when doing eurythmy later on. It is essential to devote oneself wholly to the patient and carry him with artistic warmth of heart.

As Rudolf Steiner often mentions in the course, curative eurythmy should never be used without a doctor's thorough diagnosis. The greater the collaboration with the patient's doctor the more effective the curative eurythmy will be.

REFERENCES TO THE FOURTH GERMAN EDITION

The basis for the text: The course was taken down in short-hand by the professional shorthand writer Helene Finckh (1883-1963) and then written out in longhand. The Stuttgart lecture of October 28, 1922, which is included as the eighth lecture, was probably taken down by participants. There is no shorthand report.

For the first edition (manuscript of lectures 1-6) the material was arranged by the curative eurythmist Elisabeth Baumann-Dollfus.

For the second edition (manuscript of lectures 1-6, with the addition of lecture 7) the first publication was revised by Isabella de Jaager.

For the third edition (first edition in the complete works) the publisher, Dr. Hans W. Zbinden, used Helene Finckh's original shorthand notes as a reference.

The present (fourth) edition is an unaltered impression of the third edition, the only additions being the summary of the contents and the subject index.

Concerning lectures 7 and 8:

The lecture of April 18, 1921, which was included as the seventh lecture of this course, was given in connection with the so-called second doctors' course and is contained in the volume "The Spiritual Scientific Aspect of Therapy". In that context Rudolf Steiner refers to this lecture by saying "After a short pause we shall continue by going more in the direction of eurythmy."

The lecture given in Stuttgart on October 28, 1922, and which has been included in this course as the eighth lecture, was given in connection with the "Medical Week" held in

Stuttgart from October 26-28, 1922, (see "Anthroposophical Approach to Medicine"). The lecture has been published in the present volume only, however.

How the course came about and the ladies to whom the abbreviations "Frau B. and Frl. W." refer:

Frau B. is Elisabeth Baumann-Dollfus (1895-1947) who actively participated in the development of eurythmy as from the summer of 1913. Later on she was the first eurythmy teacher at the Independent Waldorf School in Stuttgart, and she was an active member of the curative eurythmy course.

Frl. W. is Erna van Deventer, née Wolfram (1894-1976), one of the first eurythmists, and, together with Elisabeth Baumann, an active member of the curative eurythmy course. In a memorial essay of the year 1961 in the periodical "Blätter für Anthroposophie" she makes the following reference to it:

"I have two rather faded pieces of paper in front of me; one is a small drawing of the curve of Cassini and the other is a postcard dated February 1921 from Dr. Roman Boos* in Dornach. Two modest pieces of paper, and yet they are almost the only visible testimonies of the events that led up to the curative eurythmy course that Dr. Steiner gave in Dornach in the Spring of 1921 alongside the second doctors' course.

If I want to go back in memory to the time when Dr. Steiner gave the first therapeutic eurythmy exercises I have to go much further back than 1921. As early as 1915 and even earlier Dr. Steiner gave me, and probably other eurythmy teachers too, in answer to our questions, various eurythmy exercises for speaking, and hints for using in special cases we had encountered in towns all over Germany. The expression curative eurythmy did not even exist then, and Dr. Steiner called these exercises "therapeutic" eurythmy and

* Head of the Dornach administration at that time.

116

said that these arose out of the Greek Mysteries. This remark will perhaps show how earnest Dr. Steiner was even at that time about healing by means of eurythmy movements, and it will also show how deeply it was impressed upon the consciousness of us still very young teachers that "healing" is connected with "holy", and that our movements in this therapeutic eurythmy would really have to be carried by "the will to heal" if we wanted to achieve any success with this therapy. (Dr. Steiner did not coin the expression "the will to heal" until later; it was actually on the occasion of our asking him for advice, in 1923-24, whereupon he entered into our problems and gave the course for young medical students.)

Anyone who worked with Dr. Steiner in any way will remember that everything he gave was in answer to a question, a wish, or sometimes even a vague aspiration that came his way. It was the same with curative eurythmy. For instance two children with speech defects were brought to him, and he gave what we would later on have called "curative eurythmy exercises". In 1919 I met a child with curvature of the spine. Dr. Steiner entered into my questions very thoroughly and gave me the help I wanted. I could give lots more examples like this. Yet at the same time I myself was also learning, in the course of giving lessons, to observe people, and I learnt to unite the various phenomena I observed in a person, and to become aware of how many people actually in the numerous eurythmy courses round about were in need of help.

... During those years I often met Elisabeth Baumann-Dollfus, who was also one of the first eurythmists, and a deep love for the work we shared united us for many years. In 1919, after the end of the First World War, we encountered one another again when the Waldorf School was being founded. So we began to exchange our experiences, she being a teacher at the Waldorf School where she worked with Dr. Schubert's remedial class, and I being a eurythmist who in the course of the year gave eurythmy courses in almost all the big towns in Germany, and I had the privilege when I was in Stuttgart of standing in for Frau Baumann at the Waldorf School when she was ill. We each had much joy in the other, because we were aware of our common bond. We were both searching for the same thing, and what were we looking for? The *healing element* in or behind eurythmy!

This was one of the threads of destiny that bound us together. The other one was my engagement and marriage to H.A.R. van Deventer, who was himself a doctor, and who approached eurythmy from a background of medicine with the same enthusiasm that we approached medicine from a background of eurythmy. And what gave rise to it? The natural science course in Stuttgart at Christmas 1920/21.

Frau Baumann and I went to this course — more as visitors really — since we could not understand a lot of what Dr. Steiner was saying, and as eurythmists we hardly even belonged to that enlightened gathering of students and scholars! But — even if we did not understand it all with our intellect — our enthusiasm for the astronomical drawings made up for it. And one day Dr. Steiner drew something on the blackboard that made us fall on top of one another and nearly jump into the air, and that was the curve of Cassini.

This was the *external* occurrence that we needed to make us aware that the paths of the stars and the flow of forces *within* us, both sprang from the same source! For this curve of Cassini that Dr. Steiner was now describing in connection with natural science and astronomy, why, we eurythmists knew it too! As early as 1915, in the White Room of the old Goetheanum, Dr. Steiner had given four to six eurythmy teachers a series of lessons, and on this occasion he taught us "children's forms, good for children and young people from the age of three to eighty, to stop their thoughts scattering". Those were his words, and one of these forms was the curve of Cassini, to the words "We will seek one another, we feel near one another, we know one another well".

In 1915 we young people did not have the least idea why

118

he gave this form as a pedagogical exercise, in fact we hardly knew the "Why" of any of the eurythmy teaching material — and to be honest do we know it that much better today? And yet it should be our task to pass not only the exercises but also the "Why" on to our successors. The only way to do this seems to be that in the eurythmy of the future we must separate truth from error, and the source of eurythmy from a watering down of it.

This experience of "recognizing" such an apparently insignificant form was what drew me to Elisabeth Baumann and what caused her and my husband to sit together for hours discussing the problem "If this form which Dr. Steiner was illustrating in the natural science course is so important for both macrocosmic man and microcosmic man, then does not everything given us in eurythmy come from the same source, and should it not be applicable for healing?" For just as with the curve of Cassini, we had also over the years learnt about the *cosmic* and the *human* healing effect of vowels, for instance AUM. Our experience of the curve of Cassini was really only the corner-stone of the building of our surmises and experiences in the realm of eurythmy!

But how was it to be done? How were we to acquire a knowledge of "therapeutic eurythmy"? What we knew up till then — Elisabeth Baumann and I — were only small building stones that Dr. Steiner had given us on occasion. Through the fact that my husband supported us in our ideas, as a doctor — he had done quite a lot of eurythmy himself and could understand and support our endeavours from both the medical and the eurythmic side — this gave us courage to ask Dr. Steiner whilst he was still in Stuttgart whether he would like to teach us a kind of therapeutic eurythmy in a systematic way just like he had taught us ordinary eurythmy. Dr. Steiner was very kind, looked at us somewhat astonished at our bold plans, and said he would discuss the matter further with my husband in Holland, and then we would hear.

119

And thus it happened. Dr. Steiner was in Holland at the beginning of 1921, and as my husband had a strong connection with our work through his medical studies, he had a good deal of opportunity to talk with Dr. Steiner. Frau Baumann was in Stuttgart at the time and I was in Breslau, but we had both set down our wishes very clearly in writing and sent them to my husband (He was still my fiancé then). At any rate Dr. Steiner asked him one day in Holland "Do you actually have some eurythmists who would really put their backs into therapeutic eurythmy?" — to which my husband replied "Yes indeed, two at present, Frau Baumann and my future wife". "Then we can start with it" said Dr. Steiner, and instructed my husband to do the necessary organizing.

This brings me back to the beginning, for the little drawing was the "curve of Cassini" which came from an evening's discussion with Dr. Steiner, and the faded postcard from Roman Boos was his announcement from Dornach to say that the "Curative Eurythmy Course" (Dr. Steiner had now coined the name) was due to take place in Dornach at the beginning of April, along with the second doctor's course, that was also due to be given then.

In an article for the periodical "Beiträge zu einer Erweiterung der Heilkunst nach Geisteswissenschaftlichen Erkenntnissen" (1971, volume 4) headed "Curative Eurythmy: 1921-71. Its Origins, Development and Task" she describes the following:

During the second doctors' course, from April 12 to 17, 1921, Dr. Steiner gave the curative eurythmy course in six lectures, for doctors, and also for eurythmists who had been training for more than two years. Not one of us could imagine what the course would be like! Dr. Steiner stood on the platform, and Frau Baumann and I, sitting on two chairs in front of it, felt very uncomfortable, for we had instigated the situation, and in the meantime, from February till April, we had heard no word from Dr. Steiner as to how he would establish this new branch of medical science with the likes of us, who had not the slightest preparatory training in the realm of medicine!

We certainly did not have the necessary knowledge for curative eurythmy work — would it not have been much more practical and sensible for Dr. Steiner to have chosen a small group of doctors for this work? Or did Frau Baumann and I, being eurythmists, really bring something with us out of our past that seemed important to him? In the instructions he gave me shortly after the course, about the training necessary for curative eurythmy, I had my answer.

He answered our question by saying "The prerequisite for the curative eurythmy profession is that you first of all know the whole foundation of artistic eurythmy, in theory and practice. You must be capable of performing a dramatic poem on the stage, for example "der Zauberlehrling" (sorcerer's apprentice) by Goethe, and carry out all the eurythmic indications for word meaning and sentence construction, with all the forms and postures you have learnt. Not until you have mastered all the aspects of artistic eurythmy are you ready to change over to curative eurythmy. He made it clear to us that we would first of all have to master all the possibilities of artistic eurythmy, be able to find them in the cosmos as the forces of the planets and the fixed stars, then in their reflection in human speech and music, then through movements of the human body itself, and in this way we would get to know the human being, that is, ourselves, as beings who reflect macrocosm and microcosm in our own body. Not until we had grasped our situation and task would we be able to advance from the periphery of eurythmy to the centre of the healing aspect of eurythmy. Yet "first of all you must know the periphery, and then you can move on to the centre of man!" What a perspective for us, who had already been actively engaged in artistic and pedagogical eurythmy for eight years, though more in a practical way, and by learning from doing it rather than filling it with our consciousness. The vowels, consonants, parts of speech,

121

rhymes — how much more significant they now appeared to be!

...What a eurythmist should know was also clearly defined by Dr. Steiner telling me what and how I would have to learn from my husband's textbooks, the "Spalteholz"[1] and the textbook by Professor Broesicke[2] of Breslau.

Dr. Steiner told us this shortly after the curative eurythmy course, so that it was with a deep feeling of responsibility that we took our departure from Dornach.

1) Prof. W. Spalteholz of the University of Leipzig, February 1914
2) Prof. Dr. Gustav Broesicke, Breslau 1920

INDEX

A

A devotion, 59
A (effect), 20
A exercise, 19
A (for affections of the kidneys), 99
A (overcoming the animal nature), 33
Abdominal illnesses, 104
Abdominal pains, 56
Affection of the kidneys, S, A, 99
Air conditions within the organism, 99
Artistic eurythmy and curative eurythmy, 94
Astral organism (too strong or too weak), 103
Asymmetries, 101-2

B

B (function of the kidneys), 99
B (migraine), 56
B (with legs and arms), 61
Belching, 55
Breath sounds, plosive sounds, 29-30
Breathing difficulty (indistinct speaking of consonants), 20
Breathing exercises, 99

C

Centrifugal and centripetal dynamics in the organs, 99
Circulation, 55
Circulation and metabolic activity, 72-3
Circulation and thinking, 6
Circulation system warning (love E), 55
Clumsiness in walking, 102
Consolidation forces, 78
Consonants, 23
Consonants and vowels, 13, 75
Consonants for the mentally retarded, 70-2
Consonants in eurythmy, 23-4

Consonants in eurythmy, effect on the organs, 73
Consonants, luminous process, 84
Consonants, vocalic tinge, 27-8
Corpulence, 102
Curative eurythmy, 1-2, 94-5

D

D (with jump), 43
Defects (congenital), 86
Deformation, 99
Deformation (of the rhythmic system), 84
Dental process, 78
Dentals, 32
Dentition, 97-8
Dexterity, E, 56-7
Diarrhoea, 47, 104
Difference between bad standing and walking, 16
Division (into labials, dentals and palatals), 32
Drowsiness, 75
Dynamics (in the organs), 99

E

E (dexterity), 56-7
E (effect), 20
E (effect in speech), 35
E exercise, 17-18, 37
E (feeling of the sound), 17
E (love), 55
E (paralysis and abdominal illnesses), 104
E (thin people), 100-1
E (too strong or too weak an astral body), 103
Earth formation, 77
Effect of consonants, 76
Effect of consonants (guide lines), 76
Effect of vowels, 76
Egoism (and selflessness), 73

CONCERNING THE TRANSCRIPTS OF THE LECTURES

From *Rudolf Steiner, An Autobiography*, Chapter 35, 2nd Ed., Multimedia Publishing Corp., New York, 1980.

Two consequences of my anthroposophical activity are the books which were made accessible to the general public and an extensive series of lecture courses which were initially intended for private circulation and were available only to members of the Theosophical (later Anthroposophical) Society. The transcripts of the latter were taken down — some more accurately than others — during my lectures. But time did not permit me to undertake their correction. I, for my part, would have preferred spoken word to remain spoken word, but the members were in favour of private publication of the Courses. And so it came about. If I had had time to correct the transcripts, the reservation "For Members Only" need not have been made from the very first. Now it has been dropped for over a year.

Here in my autobiography it is above all necessary to explain how the two — the publications in general and in private circulation — are accommodated in my elaboration of anthrosophy.

Whoever wishes to pursue my own inner conflict and toil in my effort to introduce anthroposophy to contemporary thought, must do so with the aid of works in general circulation which include analysis of all forms of cognition of this age. Therein also lies that which crystallised within me in "spiritual vision" and from which came into existence the structure of anthroposophy, even if imperfect in many respects.

Apart from this obligation to construct anthroposophy

and thereby to serve only that which ensues when communications from the spirit world are to be transmitted to modern civilisation, the need also arose to meet the claims which were manifested within the membership as a compulsion, a yearning of the soul.

Above all, many members were greatly disposed to hearing the Gospels and the scriptural content of the Bible presented in an anthroposophical light. Courses were requested which were to examine such revelations to humanity.

Internal courses were held to meet this requirement. At these lectures only members were present who were initiated in anthroposophy. It was possible to speak to them as to those well-versed in anthroposophy. The delivery of these internal lectures was such as simply could not be communicated in written works intended for the general public.

In these closed circles I was able to discuss subjects which I would have had to present quite differently if they had been intended for a general public from the very first.

Thus in the duality of the public and private works there actually exists something of two-fold diverse origin. The wholly public writings are a result of that which struggled and toiled within me; in the private publications, the Society struggles and toils with me. I listen to the vibrations within the soul-life of the membership and within my own being and the tone of the lectures arises from what I hear there.

Nowhere has even the slightest mention of anything been made which does not proceed from the substance of anthroposophy. No concessions can be made to any prejudices or presentiments existing within the membership. Whoever reads these private publications can accept them as a true representation of anthroposophical conviction. Thus when petitions became more urgent, the ruling as to the private circulation of these publications within the membership could be amended without any hesitation. Any errors occurring in transcripts which I have not been able to revise will however have to be tolerated.

The right to pass judgment on the content of any such private publication is nevertheless reserved to those possessing the prerequisite to do so. For the great majority of these publications, this is *at least* an anthroposophical knowledge of man and the universe, in so far as its essence is presented in anthroposophy, and of "the history of anthroposophy" such as it is derived from communications from the spirit-world.

COMPLETE EDITION OF WORKS OF RUDOLF STEINER
in German, published by the Rudolf Steiner Verlag,
Dornach, Switzerland, by whom all rights are reserved.

Writings
1. Works written between 1883 and 1925.
2. Essays and articles written between 1882 and 1925.
3. Letters, drafts, manuscripts, fragments, verses, inscriptions, meditative sayings, etc.

Lectures
1. Public lectures.
2. Lectures to members of the Anthroposophical Society on general anthroposophical subjects.
   Lectures to members on the history of the Anthroposophical movement and Anthroposophical Society.
3. Lectures and courses on special branches of work:
   Art: Eurythmy, Speech and Drama, Music, Visual Arts, History of Art; Education; Medicine and therapy; Science; Sociology and the Threefold Social Order; Lectures given to workmen at the Goetheanum

The total number of lectures amount to some six thousand, shorthand reports of which are available in the case of the great majority.

Reproductions and Sketches
Paintings in water colour, drawings, coloured diagrams, eurythmy forms, etc.

When the Edition is complete the total number of volumes, each of a considerable size, will amount to several hundreds. A full and detailed Bibliographical Survey, with subjects, dates and places where the lectures were given is available. All the volumes can be obtained from the Rudolf Steiner Press in London as well as directly from the Rudolf Steiner Verlag, Dornach, Switzerland.